Afraid to Eat

Children and Teens
in Weight Crisis

■

Frances M. Berg

Edited by
Kendra Rosencrans

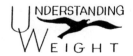
UNDERSTANDING
WEIGHT

Published by Healthy Weight Journal

Acknowledgements

I've been privileged to network with many outstanding leaders in the fields of nutrition, eating disorders, obesity, and size acceptance over the years and I thank them for their contributions to this book. My thanks to Kendra for her supurb editing, and to Ronda for her dedication and skill in putting it all together. A special thank you to my family, my husband Bert, and four children, Kathy, Rick, Cindy and Mike.

Edited by Kendra Rosencrans
Layout and production by Ronda Irwin
Cover photo by
Jon Steinbach, Steinbach Studio
Published by Healthy Weight Journal
402 South 14th Street
Hettinger, ND 58639
Tel:701-567-2646; Fax:701-567-2602.

For the first time in the history of this country, young people are less healthy and less prepared to take their places in society than were their parents.

National Commission on
Role of School and Community in
Improving Adolescent Health, 1990

Contents

Introduction

Children and teens today struggle with a major health crisis that dominates their lives in often detrimental ways. They live in a culture that tells them their bodies are wrong and promotes destructive values through media, advertising and the entertainment industries. Weight and eating issues have become an obsessive concern for American children of all ages, yet it's a crisis not being widely recognized by the health community.

This book outlines the pervasive public health problem, focusing on four aspects, their causes and detrimental effects: dysfunctional eating, eating disorders, size prejudice and overweight. It explores the social forces that have shaped these problems, such as cultural expectations and media images, and how they are intimately related. It reviews the growing body of research that documents the profound medical and psychological effects of this crisis among children and teens. It looks at the interplay of athletics, teen pregnancy, prejudice and peer pressure on these problems.

Finally, *Afraid to Eat* examines the steps educators, parents, health professionals and society need to take to help kids who struggle with these problems. It warns that children are vulnerable to the wrong kind of help and the first criteria should be to do no harm. It challenges society to protect its youth from violence, harassment, sexual abuse and stigmatization. It provides guidelines to promote the healthy growth and well-being of the whole child and every child. We must allow our children to eat without fear.

CHAPTER 1

Growing up
afraid to eat

■

America's children are afraid to eat.

It's a fear that consumes them, shattering lives, killing others. It's an obsession that dims their joy, their curiosity, their energy and their sense of what's normal.

To be overweight is to fail. It's irrational, but kids are succumbing to the same destructive cultural messages about body and weight that plague us as adults. Instead of growing up with secure and healthy attitudes about weight, eating and themselves, they're afraid of food and afraid of being fat. They believe, as do many of us, that in order to be loved, they must be thin.

Some children make unhealthy food choices and passively devote their energy to television instead of the activities of life. Others grow up hating their bodies, ridiculed by friends, adults and American culture.

It's a national public health crisis and we need to take action.

Our daughters and sons are caught — and they need us. They're not developing the eating habits, lifetime activities and self-esteem critical to becoming healthy adults with healthy weights.

This crisis consists of four major weight and eating problems, fed by our obsessions with weight and beauty — dysfunctional eating,

eating disorders, size prejudice, overweight. Some children can't eat normally. Others live with eating disorders. Some struggle with overweight. Still others fail to thrive because of the social shame they endure for being large. And we, as parents, educators, health professionals and members of society, have ignored them, punished them, and failed them.

In the 11 years I've been writing and publishing *Healthy Weight Journal*, reporting worldwide research on weight and eating issues, I've seen an astounding increase in these problems.

At first I was appalled at the disarray in the health field related to weight and eating problems, then hopeful, believing once the problems were better known they might be solved.

Eleven years have passed. It hasn't happened.

I suppose I was naive, believing that when they understood what I was seeing, health policy makers would be willing to make changes. But I underestimated the power of tradition, the marketplace, and the determination of those in power to stay their course.

Yet, these are our children, our daughters and sons, who are growing up afraid to eat, desperate to have the "right" bodies, obsessed with the need to be thin, feeling doomed if they can't measure up to perfection. They live in a world of adolescent risk, of high drug and alcohol use, violence, sexually transmitted diseases and early pregnancy, and controlling their weight and eating may seem all the more urgent.

It should come as no surprise in a country where half of adults are dieting at any one time that children see, hear and take to heart the cultural ideal that to be thin is to have the best of everything and to be fat is to fail.

These same pressures are growing worldwide, as our readers around the world assure us, but they are especially acute in the U.S.

Weight issues have become an obsessive concern for American children of all ages. Clearly it is a national crisis when harmful attempts at dieting are common in the third grade and before. It is a crisis when more than two-thirds of high school girls are dieting, one in five take diet pills, and many girls as well as boys are using laxatives, diuretics, fasting and vomiting in desperate attempts to slice their bodies as slim as they can, and when more than half our teenage girls are sadly undernourished. This is the point where our weight-obsessed culture has brought us. Our children are the innocent victims.

A need to be thin

A group of girls ages 11 to 17 were asked in one study, "If you had three wishes, what would you wish for?"

The top wish of nearly every girl was to lose weight. Not to cure cancer or save the rainforest or be a millionaire, but to be thin.

In another survey young girls said they were more afraid of becoming fat than they were of cancer, nuclear war or losing their parents.[1]

Possessed by this fear, many children don't eat normally. Some shun certain foods, others diet. There's a new name for these eating habits — they're called dysfunctional eating.

First and second graders worry about their weight. Six out of 10 high school girls diet; so do one in four high school boys. Almost every day, I hear new horror stories about how dysfunctional eating hurts children.

Teachers tell me sad stories about the meager lettuce leaves girls put on their plates in the lunch line — and how they droop, glassy-eyed in class. They tell of the school's star wrestlers, thin-faced and gaunt, who shiver in their winter jackets as they try to focus on answering a test.

Most recently, they tell me about the small girls and boys with fragile, stress-fractured bones, their growth stunted. Their young brains may be damaged as well, deprived of the fuel needed for normal development. Some children have been traumatized by radical animal rightist groups who come into their own schools and deliver deadly propaganda about the evils of eating animal foods. As a result, these kids won't eat eggs, meat or milk — the building blocks of healthy growth and development which have for generations made America's youngsters among the tallest, strongest and healthiest in the world.

I hear from parents that their college-age daughters are being taught by their classmates to eat "zero" fat — if a girl is so tempted she eats ordinary food, she must not swallow it. College girls who eat normally, or eat meat, may be harassed in their own sororities at Syracuse University in New York, says one of our subscribers, Cynthia DeTota, a registered dietitian who is the campus nutritionist.

"Your daughters will come home from college as vegetarians," one mother told me in despair.

One in 10 teens struggle with the most serious kinds of abnormal eating — potentially fatal clinical eating disorders. Some die and others are consumed by their eating disorders into college and adulthood.

When Christy Heinrich died in 1994 of anorexia nervosa, she was 22 years old and weighed 60 pounds. The Kansas City gymnast had been weight-conscious as long as she'd been competing. But in 1988, a judge at an international competition told the then 16-year-old Heinrich that she needed to watch her weight if she wanted to continue winning.

Her offending weight: 93 pounds.

One serious problem for these young people who don't eat healthily is malnutrition. Teenage girls have the poorest nutrition of any age group in the U.S. Dysfunctional eating, binge eating, fasting and dieting are disrupting their natural growth.

A recent national study revealed that the majority of girls age 11 to 19 are severely undernourished. They don't eat enough to get the calories and nutrients needed for healthy growth and development. Half are getting two-thirds or less of the Recommended Daily Allowance (RDA) of iron, calcium, vitamin A and many other essential nutrients, according to the 1995 Nutrition Monitoring report. Many girls are malnourished.[2]

Girls who are starving don't think straight.

Girls are also taking up smoking more and more as they grasp at every possible straw to lose weight. They have now caught up with boys and are smoking just as much. The Youth Risk Behavior survey shows 34 percent of high school girls and 35 percent of high school boys smoke at least monthly, and 16 percent of both girls and boys smoke more frequently.

At the same time, obesity among children and teens has skyrocketed. One in five teenagers is overweight, and the rates are higher among ethnic and racial minorities. Not only are more youngsters overweight, but they are more severely overweight than ever before. It's a complex problem with no sure-fire cure. Genetics, inactivity, and poor nutrition all play a role.

Meanwhile, large kids struggle with prejudice and stigmatization.

In 1990, a 16-year-old girl wrote to *Parade Magazine* of the anguish and humiliation she suffers because of her weight and her efforts to reduce.

"I can't speak for all fat people, but I do know that I am not lazy about losing weight. I'm always in the midst of planning a diet, in the middle of a diet or breaking a diet. I've tried sensible diets, liquid diets, crash diets," she wrote.

"I've lived my entire life with people reminding me that it isn't okay to be fat. It isn't okay to be 16 years old, 5 feet 6 inches tall, have beautiful hair and eyes, and to be fat. It isn't okay, and it isn't fair."

Body image issues are severe for young people – girls and boys.

I'm getting more letters and calls today from youngsters who seem suicidal, and it's troubling. A 17-year-old boy from California wrote me a long and anguished letter about the bulimia that is taking over his life: "There is a war going on inside me . . . I don't know what to do. It is tearing apart our family. . . I sometimes feel that death would be better than being fat and having this destroy my family."

Joelyn M., 15, sent me an E-mail message from Pennsylvania, "Can you help me? I'm a vegetarian, but mostly what I eat is lettuce. I think a lot about doing away with myself."

So I was not surprised to see the latest suicide behavior statistics from the Youth Risk Behavior Surveillance Survey. They show that more than 30 percent of high school girls and 18 percent of high school boys seriously considered suicide in the past 12 months, and 21 percent of girls and 14 percent of boys went so far as to make a suicide plan.[4]

These numbers are self-reported and may even underestimate the despair our daughters and sons are feeling. How much does this desire for self-destruction have to do with body image issues, with not measuring up, with sexual violence, harassment, being stigmatized, and the effects of self-starvation?

The shocking part of all these latest reports on malnutrition, hazardous dieting and suicide behavior is that there is no public outcry, no headlines and no public health programs to deal with these problems. The public apathy is underwhelming.

The nutrition report I quoted is more than two years old. It never hit the news — and in fact its own summary does not even mention the nutrition deficiencies it so clearly documents for teenage girls.

Ours is a society obsessed by weight. In what is surely a crime against innocence, we have set a monster loose among our children.

How can we get the monster back in the bottle?

A unifying approach

A new approach is needed to deal with these issues in healthy ways. The goal must be healthy growth and development of the whole child — his or her emotional, mental, physical, intellectual, spiritual and social development — and it must include every child of every size.

We need to help young people build self-esteem, learn assertiveness and healthy coping skills. We want them to develop their unique potential as lovable, capable, valuable individuals, and take pride in themselves and their bodies at any size, without being stigmatized.

All children deserve this.

What is needed is for people to see the big picture, to realize that the scope of today's problems includes not just overweight and its risks. It also includes eating disorders, pressures to be thin, the impact of dysfunctional eating, size prejudice and the stigmatization of large persons, women's body image issues and the failure of weight loss treatment.

The interrelatedness of these issues, encompassed in the four major problems set forth in this book, must be considered in developing health promoting approaches. Health professionals, educators and parents need to look carefully at all these problems, ever wary of the harm so easily done in the lives of vulnerable youth, and find positive ways of working together to build strengths in these areas.

The old ways of dealing with these problems haven't worked.

We must change the focus from dieting to being healthy at the weight we are. There's much evidence that keeping a stable weight through adult life is healthier than losing and gaining weight, even for large persons.

One of the most urgent needs in solving eating and weight problems is, first of all, to empower our half-starved daughters to feed themselves. The current level of malnutrition is having severe effects on their bones, growth and brain development.

Preventive programs need to be based on self-trust, with children empowered to follow their own body signals and needs. They need help in understanding that they can be healthy at the weight they are, by growing normally, and not focus on weight loss. Along with this, they need assurance of acceptance, regardless of size, shape or appearance. They need to be liberated from false and narrow images based on appearance, and taught how to evaluate and combat media stereotypes. Programs with this new approach will empower and strengthen all youngsters.

Thus, the health promoting model shown here *(figure 1)* demonstrates a unified approach based on the principles of good health for all youth at whatever size they are. The first step is to do no harm. The next is to reach toward normal eating by working on the four major problems, recognizing their interrelatedness. In this way, we will solve problems rather than create new ones. A united effort can also act on the culture in positive ways, and respond effectively to its negative pressures.

There is an underlying unity in this approach — what is healthy for the largest child in school is also healthy for the thinnest.

As the *Canadian Vitality* program stresses, living healthfully involves healthy eating, active living and positive self- and body images. It's a way of life that focuses on the quality of life in all of life.

Current confusion

The risks of focusing on one or two problems to the detriment of

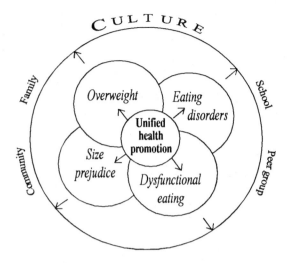

Figure 1

Health promotion approach

A unified approach focuses on good health for all children, does no harm, recognizes the interrelatedness of eating and weight problems, and strengthens the positive aspects of culture, family, friends.[1]

AFRAID TO EAT 1997

others, as in current U.S. health policy, cannot be overemphasized *(fig 2)*.

When the focus is on reducing overweight alone, there is high probability of intensifying the problems of dysfunctional eating, dangerous weight loss methods, eating disorders, and the stigmatization of larger youngsters. Today, different groups seek to solve the various problems in conflicting ways, and they give out confusing health messages. Most professionals deal with only a few elements of the problems, sometimes working at cross-purposes with others, equally well-intentioned.

Unlike obesity specialists, who sometimes focus so narrowly on making weight loss happen that they seem unaware of the consequences of their actions, eating disorder specialists are keenly aware of the dangers of promoting weight loss, but they sometimes discount the problems of excessive weight gain.

Few specialists have been willing to stand back and view the whole picture. Few have examined the broad tragic network of weight issues that holds so many lives hostage.

We need to do it now.

The crisis continues to grow. Not being effectively dealt with, the problems are acted on by the culture in ways that are often detrimental to the development of children.

Health professionals, educators and parents need to look carefully at all the problems, aware of the harm that can and is being done to vulnerable children and teens, and find positive ways of working together to build strengths in these areas.

Those who set national health policy, in particular, need to take a broader and more honest look at weight and eating problems.

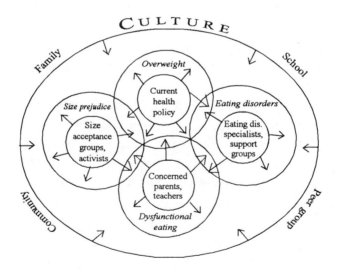

Figure 2

Current weight and eating crisis

Children are caught in a crisis in which experts, parents and others work at cross-purposes, giving out conflicting messages and allowing the negative aspects of culture to exert a more powerful influence.[2]

AFRAID TO EAT 1997

Changing their rigid stance would make a great difference, since U.S. health policy sets much of the agenda for what happens throughout the country. It also has a profound influence on how the media responds to health issues.

This nation has not dealt well with weight issues in the past. We still don't.

The traditional view, which is the official health policy view today, is that all large children and adults can and should lose weight.

Health and medical professionals who promote this view assume that any excess weight over a narrow "ideal" weight range is unhealthy, dangerous and expensive to the U.S. health system; that weight loss is always desirable and healthy for persons over "ideal" weight no matter how it is accomplished; that all large persons can successfully lose at least 10 to 15 percent of their weight and maintain it.

They further assume that publicizing the risks of obesity and stressing the importance of thinness is helping people get thin (despite all evidence to the contrary). And they fear that warning about eating disorders or the risks of weight loss may discourage people from trying to lose weight.

It is inexcusable and appalling that such fears have kept the prevention of eating disorders out of the nation's health plan in Healthy People 2000. Healthy People is the document that sets the nation's health goals for each decade. Although several goals deal with reducing obesity, none speak to the devastating prevalence of dysfunctional eating or eating disorders.

In this traditional view, it is not a concern that radical treatment methods are being prescribed for high risk patients, even children, and that underweight and normal weight youngsters are severely restricting their nutrition to lose weight. It is not a concern that smoking has increased for girls as part of their fear of fat.

Eating disorders, dysfunctional eating and size prejudice are regarded as unimportant or unrelated to any public health messages aimed at reducing overweight. It ignores the possibility that health policy itself might be contributing to these problems.

Holding this traditional view are influential leaders in federal health policy and obesity research, as well as much of the general public and health community.

It cannot be denied that many of these people have financial ties to the powerful weight loss industry, which exerts great influence in the field.

Vested interests are strong in a field like this. Thomas J. Moore charges in his book, *Lifespan,* that it is "almost impossible to find any boundary between the government, the industry and the medical elite. "He says it is "a closed circle of medical insiders operating without the normal checks and ethical barriers."

Many health officials and researchers do not share this view, however, it is the one that currently determines U.S. health policy in regard to eating and weight issues. It is a policy that exaggerates the risks of obesity and minimizes the risks of underweight, malnutrition and eating disorders. It blindly encourages weight loss above all.

Following are recent examples of this short-sighted bureaucratic policy.

- The "healthy weight" table in the 1995 *Dietary Guidelines for Americans* sets a new standard for thinness. It removes the 10 to 15 pound 1990 age allowance after age 35, despite strong evidence that a wider range is healthy, especially for women and as people grow older. All adults with a body mass index of 25 or over, or who have gained 10 pounds since they reached adult height, are told bluntly, "You need to lose weight." The guidelines are published every five years on order of Congress by the US Departments of Agriculture and Health and Human Services.[5]

- "Almost any of the commercial weight-loss programs can work," declares a consumer brochure by WIN (Weight-control Information Network) — despite providing no credible evidence for this at all. WIN is an arm of the National Institute of Diabetes & Digestive & Kidney Disease and seems aimed at keeping up consumers' and clinicians' flagging interest in weight loss treatment. The WIN newsletter publicizes the short-term successes of weight loss treatments as if important, and often discounts research on weight loss failure. (Choosing a safe and successful weight-loss program, WIN, NIDDK.)

■ Weight cycling, or yo-yo dieting, was claimed to be harmless in a special report of selectively presented research, despite a considerable body of evidence to the contrary, by the National Task Force on Prevention and Treatment of Obesity, a federal advisory group for NIDDK. The report urges people not to let concerns over weight cycling deter them from efforts to lose weight. This shaky report is promoted and referenced heavily by the diet industry, the Task Force and WIN.[7]

■ *Weighing the Options,* a 1995 book that evaluates the available weight loss programs, basically finds all weight loss methods safe and effective, and seems to suggest that more people undergo gastric surgery to reduce. The book defines long-term weight loss as a period of just one year, but this one-year "follow-up" can begin on sign-up day and apparently include six months or more of weight loss. This, despite the fact the American Heart Association says weight loss is not long term unless maintained for at least five years, and virtually all studies show continued regain does not stop after one year. *Weighing the Options* is published by the Institute of Medicine, National Academy of Sciences, a nonprofit group chartered by Congress to advise the federal government on health policy.[7]

Groups like these are pressing to launch a major campaign in schools to teach kids the risks of overweight, screen for weight, and get large children on weight loss programs. And they are working hard to get insurance companies to pay for weight loss treatment for both children and adults.

The truth is that we do not have any safe and effective method of weight loss treatment, even with the new prescription diet pills, and our health and medical specialists should stop pretending that we do.

It's time to confess we don't know the answers. Time to stop pretending and get serious about solving weight problems instead of letting the media, advertising, and the entertainment and diet industries lead us into deeper trouble.

Other health problems and diseases are approached honestly, in a straight-forward manner. No one has pretended cancer is cured, then worked secretly backwards to see what went wrong with the cure. We haven't burdened heart patients with the onus of curing themselves.

Miracle cures

Over the last 15 years reporting on the subject, and attending national and international conferences, I've watched a steady stream of miracle cures come and go.

I was there when John Garren introduced his Garren-Edwards stomach balloon, overwhelmed by the enthusiasm of admiring physicians, and a few years later, at a Harvard meeting as he stood alone by his posters, looking forlorn and rejected, his hastily-granted FDA approval withdrawn.

No matter. Attention, enthusiasm and admirers by now clustered around promoters of the very-low-calorie diets (800 or less calories) with their "amazing, miracle" results.

I knew Dr. Peter Lindner, one of the great diet doctors of the 1980s, who coauthored with George Blackburn, MD, of Harvard, one of the initial studies that "proved" the success of very-low-calorie diets using safer liquid formulas than those that caused numerous deaths in the 1970s. Theirs became a classic oft-quoted study that gave much of impetus to the liquid diet's soaring second wave of "miracles," which again ended disastrously.

Lindner was a magician and cheerleader, urging on his patients and colleagues alike with great enthusiasm. He had scores of grateful patients, and I feel sure his motivation was to help them.

Then why did he grow increasingly despondent? His friend told me it was because, as he confessed before he died, he made a five-year check of his former patients, and not one of them — not one — had kept off for five years any of the weight they lost.

Still, by then his study had taken on a life of its own. It was referenced, quoted and followed up by hundreds, probably thousands, of nearly identical studies "proving" the success of VLCDs. These are still being presented at scientific conferences and published in scientific journals.

After liquid diets (even now in their failure being replaced by a very-low-calorie diet called, oddly, the protein-sparing fast because it contains some real food and supposedly, although this is not true, spares the dieter's muscles), came Slim Fast and its imitators that filled grocery aisles for a couple of years. Then thigh cream. Now again, diet pills.

It has been my mission to investigate and report the truth about these miracle cures.

One cult after another, as one scientist complained.

And these are just the legal, medically-sanctioned cures. We've reported on some two hundred fraudulent products besides: earrings, appetite patches, hypnosis, body wraps, vacuum pants, battery-operated belts, herbal teas, soap, cookies, "mushrooms," starch blockers, cure-all pills, drinks to detoxify the body. Many have killed. I get heartbreaking calls from victims' families.

It's been a circus.

Except for its victims. And when the victims are children, it's especially hard to bear.

Meanwhile, the one method that can work and does no harm — gradually changing to a more moderate way of eating, living more actively and relieving stress — is steadfastly ignored. There's no profit in it.

Current health policy has lost much support among educators and health professionals. For many, it runs counter to their experience in working with weight reduction and, knowing the high failure rates, they refuse to collude in putting more pressure on large people.

Further, several candid reports from the National Institutes of Health and the National Center for Health Statistics recently have warned that most people who lose weight by any method regain the weight they lost, and that adequate studies of safety and effectiveness are not available for any of these methods.[8]

It's clear that the traditional paradigm needs to be replaced by one that helps children and does not harm them.

We must allow our children to eat without fear.

CHAPTER 2

Our culture fails
to nurture its youth

■

Modern culture is youth-centered, yet in many ways it does not provide an environment that is nurturing or supportive for the healthy growth and development of our children and youth. In fact, it nurtures serious problems.

This is especially true for girls, which is probably the reason their suicide behavior rates are double those of boys in every category.

"A girl-poisoning culture . . . a girl-destroying place," psychologist Mary Pipher brands our society, even in Nebraska, in her book, *Reviving Ophelia.*

Pipher says that in early adolescence girls are expected to sacrifice the parts of themselves that our culture considers masculine on the altar of social acceptability. They have to shrink their souls down to petite size.

Lookism, appearance and above all, thinness, are the criteria by which girls are judged. Even magazines for teenage girls give training in lookism. The emphasis is on makeup, fashion, weight and how to attract boys, with almost no space given to sports, hobbies or careers.

What young people want most is to belong, to be accepted. They are always searching, trying out and learning by trial and error. Culture, family, community and friends show them the way. But today family and community are losing out to the stronger influence of pop culture, the entertainment industry and peer group pressure. The messages they get about how to belong and be accepted are often confusing, conflicting and detrimental to their well-being.

Pipher sees the culture as splitting adolescent girls into true and false selves — one that is authentic and one culturally scripted. They can be authentic and honest, or they can be loved and admired. Girls fight to preserve their wholeness and authenticity, but most choose to be socially accepted, take up false selves, and abandon their true selves. In public they become who they are supposed to be.

Girls struggle with mixed messages, "Be beautiful, but beauty is only skin deep. Be sexy, but not sexual. Be honest, but don't hurt anyone's feelings. Be independent, but nice. Be smart, but not so smart that you threaten boys."

The issues girls struggle with are barely discussed, certainly not in the teen magazines they read or the television shows they watch.

We can help to strengthen girls, encourage emotional toughness and self-protection, support and guide them, but Pipher says the important thing is to change our culture.

"We can work together to build a culture that is less complicated and more nurturing, less violent and sexualized and more growth-producing. Our daughters deserve a society in which all their gifts can be developed and appreciated."

Boys, too, are bewildered by their perceptions of what our culture expects of them. They live in a culture that showcases men as glamourous "macho" figures yet demands equality, that flaunts sexuality but fears to discuss it, where they are goaded by friends to harass and exploit girls, and where the girls they know are obsessed with their bodies, eating and weight, and can talk of little else. Like their sisters, many are emerging from a childhood of trauma, violence or sexual abuse.

How thin is thin enough?

Television, movies and other social media probably have the strongest and most dangerous influence on children. At no time in history has the cultural obsession with thinness been more severe. What's it doing to children, particularly girls? Is it sabotaging forever their chances for healthy weight, healthy self-esteems and healthy, productive lives?

Studies show that teens today get their values more from the media and friends than from family or community. Both boys and girls are being taught that only thin people are worthy of love, attention and success. They turn that expectation on themselves and their friends, dieting to meet it, hating when they don't.

It seems to me — and I've been watching — that women on television are thinner this year than last, and that last year they were thinner than the year before. Often now they show us their thin, wispy bodies from the side so we can get a good look at how narrow they really are, back to front.

It breaks my heart to see a line-up of thin girls from the side — as with high school basketball cheerleaders, their stomachs caved in, bony clavicles and hip bones protruding. Where are the bodies they have worked so hard to perfect? There's no body, only bones, arms, legs, hair and that frightening skeletal face, screaming out cheers — or maybe, screaming for help from us adults who have abandoned them.

The cultural lesson: Thin is in, fat is out.

Advertising is a $130 billion industry and the most powerful educational force in America. It has designed the cultural ideals of the late 20th century. "Each era has exacted its own price for beauty, though our era is unique in producing a standard based exclusively on the bare bones of being, which can be disastrous for human health, happiness and productivity," says Roberta Seid, PhD, of the University of Southern California.

Here's how *Newsweek* recently described "the look" of the late 1990s:

"It is a slimmer, more dissipated vision. . . reedy, women with hollow curves and sinewy lines. . . small, frail-looking. . . wan and disengaged. . . austere as the times. . . human coat hangers. . . Clothes fall off them."[1] These images have toppled the "curvaceous supermodels" of the past decade. It's a "return to reality. . . down to earth." The magazine concludes this proves that "men and their appetites" don't rule the world.

Seid writes that in the past, excesses of fashion were severely criticized by social authorities, including doctors, teachers, clergy, parents and feminists. Moralists stressed that there were values more important than outward appearance.

But no more. "In the late 20th century all these authorities, especially physicians, seemed to agree that one could never be too thin."[2]

The lookism message is sold thousands of times per day, through television and movies and magazines and billboards and newspapers and songs. To girls, the command is be thin, avoid fat and live a wonderful life. To boys, it becomes a command to build muscle, sculpt, become the ultimate muscle man — or you won't be worthy.

It's a success. Media pressure to be thin is stronger now than at any time in the last 19 years, according to a recent study that compiled statistics for television commercials on diet foods, diet program foods and chemically-based reducing aids, using advertising data from the *Network Television Books*.[3]

Diet promotions, non-existent in 1973, now comprise about 5 percent of TV advertisements. The trend continues to grow, expanding into other media.

Jean Kilbourne, EdD, author of *Still Killing Us Softly: Advertising and the Obsession with Thinness*, argues that advertising overpowers almost every other cultural message through sheer force. The average American sees 1,500 ads per day and spends a year and a half of a lifetime watching TV commercials.

"The tyranny of the ideal image makes almost all of us feel inferior," Kilbourne says. "We are taught to hate our bodies, and thus learn to hate ourselves. This self-hatred takes an enormous toll. . . (in) feelings of inferiority, anxiety, insecurity, and depression."

The ideal body, the ideal myth

The ideal female body type is now at the thinnest 5 percent of a normal weight distribution, say feminist writers. This excludes 95 percent of American women. A statistical deviation has been made to seem the norm, with millions of women believing they are abnormal or "too fat." This mass delusion causes enormous suffering for women and becomes a prison for many, even though it sells a lot of products.[4]

"For women to stay at the official extreme of the weight spectrum requires 95 percent of us to infantilize or rigidify to some degree our mental lives," says Naomi Wolf, author of *The Beauty Myth.*

The increasing pressures to be thin and their reflection in cultural images are vividly illustrated by a 30-year survey of Miss America contestants and *Playboy* magazine centerfold girls from 1959 to 1988. These women — cultural icons — have become thinner each year. Now the typical contestant or model weighs in at 13 percent to 19 percent below expected weight.

The clinical criteria for anorexia nervosa is 15 percent below expected weight. To drop weight further is to risk death by starvation, say researchers.[5]

"Pathologically underweight women are being held up as cultural ideals," says David Greenfeld, MD, medical director of the Yale-New Haven Hospital Adolescent and Young Adult Treatment Unit.[6]

Young Olympic gymnasts, the role models of many girls, are becoming younger, smaller and much thinner.[7] The champions in the winner's circle are often 16 or younger, weigh less than 90 pounds and are 4 feet, 10 inches or shorter. Body fat levels are under 10 percent.

I felt somewhat more hopeful watching the 1996 Olympic games in Atlanta. These gymnasts were older — almost the women athletes we've been hoping for — then I heard the tiny, piping, child-like voice of the injured 17-year-old. Was she almost a woman? I don't think so.

Even children's books reflect and repeat the Western obsession with thinness. One study found that illustrations of young girls have portrayed them progressively thinner over the past 80 years, while no consistent trend was evident for young boys.[8]

Thin lesson teaches self-hate

"Because our society is so focused on appearance, body image becomes central to our feelings of self-esteem and self-worth, overshadowing qualities and achievements in other aspects of our lives," says Merryl Bear, coordinator of the National Eating Disorder Information Centre in Toronto, Ontario.

"This cultural focus on looking a particular way is taught. Today, being slender has come to have other meanings attached, such as being seen to be in control of one's self and one's life, successful, self-disciplined and attractive."[9]

There are three ways the media creates a distorted picture of reality which adversely affects girls and women, says Karin Jasper, PhD, of the Women's Center Toronto.[10] She says the false messages contribute to the prevalence of eating disorders.

In portraying women, food and weight issues, the media distorts reality by (1) frequently propagating myths and falsehoods, (2) normalizing or even glamorizing what is abnormal or unhealthy, and (3) creating the false impression that all women are alike by failing to represent whole segments of the real world.

Girls and boys believe it, react to it.

Advertising expertly conveys the message to kids that you're not okay — and here's what you need to do to fix what's wrong.

High school girls say they are terrified of being overweight. In a study of 326 New York high school girls, 72 percent said they had tried to diet. About half the girls were of normal weight, 36 percent were underweight, 17 percent were overweight. Yet, 20 percent of underweight girls, 32 percent of normal weight girls and 54 percent of overweight girls said they were dieting.[11]

Leslie Morgan describes how "weight hate" has become a part of the American female identity in an article in *Seventeen* magazine. She calls it an insidious form of self-loathing that is reinforced everywhere a girl goes.[12]

Girls talk about how they look — and how much they hate how they look — on the bus to school, between math and history class, during lunch, after school, when they shop on the weekend. They think about the "cellulite" on their legs, their fat thighs, their not-flat-enough stomach all day long — whether they're on a diet or not, whether they "need" to be on a diet or not. It's an unquestioned part of their life, and it dictates how they feel about themselves and colors how they feel about everything

Kris Adler of Bala-Cynwyd, Pa., is a 15-year-old girl who is "pretty, smart, very perceptive," happy at home and has lots of friends. She is normal weight "even slim," but obsessed with her body. Adler tells Morgan her story.

"Every day at school at least one freshman girl comes up to me and tells me I have a great body," she explains. "But I weigh myself three times a day so that the scale doesn't creep up. It should be creeping down. It's not so much that I think I'm fat, it's just that I'd like to take some flesh from one part of my body and put it in other places.

"If I weighed five pounds less I'd be closer to perfect. I'd respect myself more."

Boys are also affected today by pressures to shape their bodies to match current perfectionist ideals. They are increasingly being targeted by fitness, muscle and body sculpting magazines and products. Body dissatisfaction is becoming the focus of advertising directed toward males as it has been for females. The value being taught: Only physical perfection is acceptable — you must keep trying.

As boys take in this message, they're responding. Several community studies have reported alarmingly high prevalence of severe weight concerns and unhealthy eating habits among male students.

Eating disorder specialists I know tell me they are seeing many more boys with eating disorders, recently. They blame some of this on the proliferation of muscle magazines telling boys how to get their bodies right.

One study of 321 students, age 12 to 19, found 2.4 percent of the boys along with 15 percent of girls had eating disorder-like symptoms. These boys were at the lower end of the weight range considered normal. They had serious concerns about eating and body shape, even though their concerns were not as serious as those of girls.[13] Boys who don't think they measure up or who are unhappy with their fatness often struggle with dieting and weight loss in much the same way as girls. However, studies suggest that the body concerns of most boys focus on building up lean body mass, and "sculpting" their muscles, rather than reducing.   This can lead them into extreme forms of exercise and body building. Some specialists see this as acting out a defense against conflict-laden concerns, often around the age of puberty, an overwhelming sense of insecurity, separation fears, boundary uncertainty, and specific sexual identity fears. The emotional issues are expressed as extreme body dissatisfaction and an intense desire to change it.[14]

Still, weight obsession and dieting in young men is far less prevalent than it is in young women — as are eating disorders and the destruction of self-worth.

"How easily weight obsession is dismissed as an inevitable phase of female development," charges Susan Wooley, PhD, professor of psychology at the University of Cincinnati. "Would things be different if our hospitals and clinics were filled with young men whose educations and careers were arrested by the onset of anorexia nervosa, bulimia, or the need to make dieting and body shaping a full-time pursuit?"

We may get the chance to find out.

Body, identity crises

By age 2, girls are watching television and starting their daily exposure to messages that show women who are successful are thin. As preschoolers, they are already hearing that certain types of foods, especially sugar, might make them "fat." Of course, they are also seeing and hearing their mothers, teachers, older sisters, and women in general objectify, distrust, and battle their bodies in order to make them acceptably thin.

Six-year-olds understand that fat is undesirable, and many know that people who want to lose weight can diet and exercise. Most important, a substantial minority of elementary school girls are concerned about their body shapes and have already tried to lose weight at least once. By fourth grade, 40 percent or more of girls "diet" at least occasionally. Those who do not are gathering information and forming values and opinions about body shape and weight management.

Weight preoccupation and body dissatisfaction is occurring earlier and earlier. Forty percent of girls and 25 percent of boys in grades 1 through 5 in an Ohio study reported trying to lose weight. About twice as many girls (25 percent) as boys reported restricting or altering their food intake.

In this study, girls who were trying to lose weight seemed more distressed about their shape than nondieting girls, as did dieting boys compared with nondieting boys. Dieting children tended to be heavier, had lower body self-esteem, and greater levels of dissatisfaction with their weight and shape than children with no history of trying to lose weight. However, at this early stage the majority of children did not mention thinness as important to attractiveness.[15]

But in a study of 5th graders, University of South Carolina researchers found more than 40 percent of these children felt too fat or wanted to lose weight, even though 80 percent were not overweight. They found children as young as age 9 had severe eating disorders, including anorexia nervosa and bulimia nervosa. The researchers suggest this bodes trouble ahead.[16]

One-third of the girls in a rural Iowa survey of over 400 fourth graders said they "very often worried about being fat" and nearly half of the girls "very often wished they were thinner." About 40 percent of the children dieted "sometimes or very often." Twice as many girls as boys expressed concerns about their size or weight. Some of these may be laying the foundation for eating disorders. Yet, even dieting and body dissatisfaction falling short of clear eating disorders warrant concern, warn the researchers.[17]

By contrast, the African American culture seems to define beauty by more than body size. There seems to be room for women of many sizes, and black girls learn that they don't have to be thin to be beautiful. An Arizona study that compared ideals of beauty for 300 adolescent girls found that rigid and fixed images held by white girls contrasts sharply with the more flexible beauty images of African American girls.

Most of the white girls were dissatisfied with their bodies and wanted to lose weight as a way to be popular and "perfect." Over 90 percent were dissatisfied with their weight even when it was normal. Almost as one they described their "perfect girl." She weighed 120 pounds, had very long legs and long blonde hair. Comparing themselves to this ideal, the girls were dissatisfied with their weight and appearance. Perversely, these girls did not support their peers who were closest to this ideal, but felt envious and competitive with them. The younger girls in early adolescence were most severely affected by these kinds of self-defeating images.

In contrast to this, the African American girls held images of beauty which were flexible, fluid and unrelated to a particular size. They were based on each girl's sense of self, style, confidence, and "looking good." Looking good meant that a girl was projecting her self-image, establishing a presence, creating and presenting a sense of style, and "making what you have work for you." These girls said they were supported in their efforts to "look good" by other girls and by family, friends and community.[18]

Black girls in the Youth Risk Behavior survey were dieting at about two-thirds the rates of white and Hispanic girls, and their suicidal behavior was only about two-thirds as high.

Famous role models

Mary Evans Young describes what body image issues have meant for four famous women, two British and two American — all role models for adolescent girls. She says their treatment by the media and the public regarding their size, shape and weight, serve to remind all girls and women that their bodies are open to comment, and that any deviation carries the risk of public disapproval.[19]

● Princess Diana. Before marriage, Diana is wearing a long, flowing, semi-transparent skirt and holding a child in the famous photograph. She is "probably a size 12." The public received no information about her skills or her work but a great deal about her looks and what she wore, reminding others that a woman's appearance is how she'll be judged. In the subsequent glare of the media, the press hounded Princess Diana as she lost weight, her hair became blonder, and she grew image-conscious. Once Diana lost too much weight for the media. "There was mock concern" when it was suspected that she might be suffering from anorexia or bulimia. She was criticized for playing with her food and for her faddish eating. "Diana had gone too far . . . she couldn't win. It was a pointed reminder to all of us that our margin of acceptability is very narrow and non-negotiable, and that failure invites a heavy penalty."

● Sarah Ferguson. Before her marriage to Prince Andrew, there is an early impression of Sarah: "She had just finished a day's work at a publishing firm and was happily skipping along, smiling at the photographers and film crews . . . wearing a gathered, calf-length skirt and a navy blue top, probably a dress size 12-14. She looked so ordinary and so happy . . . . a living contradiction of the "thin" edict — she had escaped the tyranny."

But as Young tells it, the press soon started to pull Sarah apart, criticizing her size and shape, her hairstyles, her dress sense. Sarah seemed to reel, and there followed a well-publicized array of exercise and reducing scenes. While the world watched, the new princess turned into a thin and very different person. But her new, waif-like figure did not insure a happy marriage. She has since regained much of that weight and is again a target for comments about her size and shape, while Andrew largely escapes hurtful comments about his size."

● Elizabeth Taylor. Over 30 or 40 years, in countless pictures and articles the press has chronicled Liz Taylor's relationship with food, dieting, fat farms and up and down cycles of weight. "A photograph of a 'fallen star' — which means 'fat' — fetches a premium price in the press. So long as she is thin, we will all want and love her . . . and aspire to be like her. This message is not lost on ordinary women. Already feeling a bit insecure, we know we need to be loved."

● Oprah Winfrey. If ever we needed an example of the way women are tyrannized into being thin, Oprah Winfrey is that example, says Young. She has lost weight, regained, lost again, regained, and shared with the public her experiences, successes and failures around food, weight and size. Oprah is a warm, caring, compassionate woman who has accomplished much, yet has said her greatest achievement was losing weight.

Young asserts that the treatment received by famous women like these "serves to chastise and tyrannize the rest of us." It is a reminder that women are targets for being sized up in a way that brings other girls and women into line.

For women, she says, "Our bodies are perceived as public property — up for scrutiny and debate, rather than a personal matter. Because we all have to be very thin, it stands to reason that the fatter ones amongst us will be pressured most. I believe that if we accept that even one woman should be oppressed for her body size and shape we are all oppressed by body size and shape — because that is the gauge by which we are all being measured."

Alicia Silverstone, a slim teenage movie star of Batman fame, was ridiculed in the press when she attended the 1996 Academy Awards, because she had gained five or 10 pounds since making her last movie (for which she probably lost weight). Headlines read "Batman and Fatgirl," and "Look out Batman, here comes Buttgirl." She was called "More Babe than Babe."

Silverstone's director asked, "What did this child do? Have a couple of pizzas? The news coverage was outrageous, disgusting, judgmental and cruel!"

What messages does this send to other young women? Will it keep them in line, dieting and starving? Will Silverstone be more careful next time about being seen in public between diets?

Other messages in the mix

When Sprite launched a marketing campaign for a new diet soda, the company chose a bony girl listlessly nursing her diet drink and boasted in the advertisement that her nickname was "Skeleton." The company pulled the ad in response to public protest.

"There's something very sick going on here," said the mother of an anorexic daughter in a Boston consumers group that boycotted Diet Sprite as a result of the ad.

There is a cultural sickness when emaciated, vulnerable, passive, childlike females are idealized as role models.

The thin ads also send other messages to girls. Take the recent Calvin Klein ads that feature thin, vulnerable, childlike waifs in sexually provocative poses. Other ads show models as young, wistful and sexually alluring, doing nothing at all but displaying themselves while males reinforce ownership of them by towering over or grasping them, says Esther Rothblum, PhD, professor of psychology at the University of Vermont.[20]

Those cultural messages potentially promote child sexual abuse, which is often linked to eating disorders, some researchers say.

Barbie — one of the most enduring cultural icons for girls — has body proportions that can't exist in reality: tiny waist, large breasts, long legs and long, stately neck. Yet she has thighs that never rub together, "big" hair, feet deformed from constantly wearing high heeled shoes, and outfits and accessories that glorify and promote self-absorption, primping, exhibitionism and materialistic behavior.

"What better way to ensure an constant supply of these decorative, nonactivist women than to train little girls to emulate this look and attitude very early age?" asks Lynn Meletiche, a size-activist, in the NAAFA Newsletter. "How better, than by giving them a sample, in the form of a Barbie — and all her attendant accessories, to serve as a constant reminder of the look and attitude they are expected to achieve?"[21]

These attitudes will likely influence the way these girls interpret and react to pubertal changes, say Linda Smolak and Michael Levine, professors of psychology at Kenyon College in Gambier, Ohio.[22]

With nearly all the messages about thinness aimed at girls and women, some researchers see strong ties between the American public health crisis over weight and eating disorders and an intentional cultural oppression of women. The attack messages work best when the target is young.

"I am deeply concerned about what is happening to young girls in our society today," says Paula Levine, PhD, former president of Eating Disorders Awareness and Prevention. "Young girls up until the age of 11 are confident, unafraid of conflict, and willing to say exactly what is on their minds. As they enter puberty, however, they adjust to society's messages about what young women are 'supposed' to be — nice, kind, caring, self-sacrificing, agreeable, and compliant."

In classrooms across the country, girls are encouraged to speak quietly, defer to boys, avoid math and science classes, and to value popularity and appearance over integrity and intelligence.

"If it is true that by the time young girls in this country reach puberty, they are voiceless, their self-esteem is at a low ebb, and they feel anxious, inferior and out of control, is there any more fertile ground for the development of an eating disorder? I think not."

Levine says that these girls need to recapture the time in their lives when they were confident, courageous, and critical thinkers.

"Only when they begin to value themselves as worthy human beings and not as objects of beauty will we begin to win the war on eating disorders."[23]

Setting the stage

But the odds against that are incredibly high.

"'Why are so many girls in therapy in the 1990s?'' asks Pipher in her book, *Reviving Ophelia*. Because, she answers, "they are coming of age in a more dangerous, sexualized and media-saturated culture. They face incredible pressure to be beautiful and sophisticated, which in junior high means using chemicals and being sexual. As they navigate a more dangerous world, girls are less protected."

Yet, this is happening at a time when women have more freedom and independence than ever before. They can command companies, lead hospitals, hold public office and make millions.

Who is pressuring women to be abnormally thin (and men as well, to a lesser extent), and why? And, most critically: How does this pressure affect young girls and children of all sizes? How does it affect girls with eating disorders? What about boys and young men?

Girls have never had more opportunities to develop their minds, yet they grow up feeling as though their bodies were being constantly watched. They learn to feel disconnected from their bodies, as if they are disembodied, observing themselves from the outside, say these experts.

"Girls do not simply live in their bodies but become aware of how their bodies appear in the eyes of boys . . . By seeing their own bodies as images in boys eyes, they begin to observe rather than to experience their own bodies; their bodies become 'Other' to themselves," say Deborah Tolman, EdD, and Elizabeth Debold, MEd, of Harvard University.[24]

Some are asking: What is "normal" and what is "disordered," for girls growing up in a culture that forces them to live as if their bodies are being "watched, desired and judged?" A culture that encourages girls to use "the power of weakness"; that allows high rates of violence and sexual assault on women, at the same time it demands the female body be highly attractive?

Some experts are calling these demands a crime against our children, a monster. "The public conscience is fast asleep," says Naomi Wolf, author of *The Beauty Myth*. The public is silent when young women die, she adds.[25]

Is it about women's freedom?

Why is this gaunt stereotype so persistently promoted and the diversity of real women ignored?

From a feminist perspective, the selling of thinness is seen as a manipulative tool to prevent women from gaining power in the work force. This travesty is not being perpetuated on women by individual men who after all have female friends, lovers, wives, sisters, daughters, but by the political power structure and multinational corporations bent on shaping women into the ultimate consumers, perennially dissatisfied with their appearance, says Wolf.

In a searing account, Wolf charges that this power structure, acting largely through the media, especially women's magazines and their advertisers, unite to force women into a competition of continual striving for thinness and beauty. It's a cruel struggle they can't win.

In this struggle, every girl and woman is made to feel a failure in her attempts to perfect her body and face. No matter what her successes in other areas of life, she falls short. Further, she feels that her body is constantly on display and being judged unfavorably.

Wolf also points out that the adverse effects of self starvation, in the quest for a thin body, keeps women weak, preoccupied, passive, and off track from career ambitions.

Dieting and thinness began to be female preoccupations when women got the vote around 1920. Never before had there been idealized "the look of sickness, the look of poverty, and the look of nervous exhaustion."

The new, leaner form replaced the more curvaceous one with startling rapidity, Wolf says. It was a great weight shift that must be understood as one of the major historical developments of the century. It was a direct solution to the threat posed by the women's movement and her newly-won economic and reproductive freedom.

"Prolonged and periodic caloric restriction is a means to take the teeth out of this revolution. . . so that women just reaching for power would become weak, preoccupied, and mentally ill in useful ways and in astonishing proportions," said Wolf.

A cultural fixation on female thinness is not an obsession about female beauty but an obsession about female obedience, Wolf charges. It's "about how much social freedom women are going to get away with or concede." Girls are still being admonished to keep their place, not to strive too hard to compete.

The "good girl" today is the thin girl, the one who keeps her appetite for food (and for power, sex and equality) under control, says Kilbourne.

Sexual harassment

Three Canadian researchers think sexual harassment may be one of the important ways in which young girls learn to feel shame, embarrassment, rejection and hatred toward their developing bodies. June Larkin, Carla Rice and Vanessa Russell, Women's Studies specialists at the University of Toronto, organized focus groups in schools in which girls recorded in their journals and shared incidents of sexual harassment.

They suggest that sexual harassment (or "teasing") is a tool of oppression that can alienate girls from their developing bodies and give them a distorted sense of self.

"We have heard countless accounts of this contempt being expressed by their male peers: the girl who is afraid to walk home from school because she is forced to walk past a gang of adolescent boys who routinely call her a "fat bitch" while they pelt her with stones; the girls who do not want to walk down a certain hallway in their high school because they are afraid of being publicly rated on a scale of one to 10 and coming out on the low end; the girls who are subjected to barking, grunting and mooing calls and labels of 'dogs,' 'cows,' or 'pigs' when they pass by groups of male students; those who are teased about not measuring up to the buxom, bikini-clad girls that drape the pages of various newspapers; and the girls who are grabbed, pinched, groped and fondled as they try to make their way through the school corridors."

Having to ward off comments about being "as flat as the walls," or "a carpenter's dream" created among many of the girls a growing uneasiness about their developing bodies. A young girl's body image is developed through the messages she receives about her body, her own perception of her body, and her resulting feelings about her body.

As one girl summed it up, "I feel bad about my body and I wish I was a boy."

The Toronto researchers charge that harassing words thrown at girls do not slide harmlessly away as the taunting sounds dissipate. "They are slowly absorbed into the child's identity and developing sense of self, becoming an essential part of whom she sees herself to be. Harassment involves the use of words as weapons to inflict pain and assert power. Harassing words are meant to instill fear, heighten bodily discomfort, and diminish the sense of self."

Sexual harassment is so commonplace it is often perceived as normal, an integral part of female development, and gets largely ignored. Yet it is one of the more pervasive ways that teenage girls are reminded of the hazards of living within a woman's body. Larkin, Rice and Russell see harassment as a pervasive form of violence that contributes to young women's uneasiness about their bodies and results in a disruption of healthy female development.[26]

Sexual harassment may be one of the most important ways in which young girls' "excitement about their developing bodies is crushed," according to Larken, Rice and Russell. It's a process that brands girls as defective, inferior, and inadequate.

Stigmatizing girls who don't measure up in body shape or appearance is a way of marking them as different, defining that difference as inferior, and using it to justify oppression, they point out. The rejection is experienced by the entire peer group, both boys and girls. Stigmatizing large girls also becomes a way to keep thinner girls in line, continuing to focus on diet and restricting their food.

Oppression can take many forms.

Harassment, sexual violence, and stigmatization are three interrelated ways that a girl's resources are weighed down, leading to eating and body struggles, say Larkin, Rice and Russell.

Sexual abuse

Sexual violence is the most graphic and oppressive tool for subordinating women, they point out. Often girls report they use bingeing and purging as a way of expelling the frightening feelings that come from being sexually traumatized. They may develop eating and weight struggles, cutting and burning themselves, or dissociating with their body as a way of disconnecting from the source of their vulnerability. Rape, incest or sexual abuse in childhood is reported by 30 to 40 percent of women, they suggest.

In the traditional view of eating disorders, until the late 1980s, sexual abuse has been discounted in much the way it was disavowed by Sigmund Freud in the 19th century in his treatment of "hysterical" women. The field of eating disorders, its conference reporting, and journal publishing was dominated by men who refused to take it seriously.

It's about shame

The consequence of all this is shame, often felt as the result of humiliation and failure to measure up to high standards of appearance. Shame is the response to being violated, harassed and stigmatized, the overwhelming sense of being inadequate and wrong. Shame as a result of harassment and oppression can make girls want to disappear, become invisible, to disconnect from their bodies while engaging in "relentless body criticism and improvement in an effort to bolster their shattered self-esteem," say the Toronto specialists.

Rice says this can make girls vulnerable to chronic dieting and eating disorders, "For someone faced with unrelenting discrimination in the form of blatant public hostility and disgust, demeaning and dehumanizing jokes, and unwanted advice . . . losing weight becomes an attractive means of attempting to retrieve lost self-esteem as well as gaining and achieving success."

Girls who stop eating when boys call them "cows" or "pigs," thus may be striving for approval and self-respect by trying to create a more acceptable body, rather than engaging in pathological practices.

Girls shut down

Girls' growing preoccupation with their bodies as they move into adolescence has been interpreted as expressing their need for male approval. But feminist writers suggest this may be more about girls' need for self-protection and having some power.

The Toronto writers say ogling by males quickly teaches girls the risks inherent in their maturing bodies. They find leering can be a process used by males to select those females who will be the target of their future sexual and abusive comments and behavior.

They quote Marian Botsford Fraser, "At some point in their physical development, all female children lose the protection of baby fat and barrettes and become prey in a game in which there are rules only if the laws are broken . . . The worst messages come from men. I have watched the way that grown men feel free to look at young girls . . . lets his eyes slide all over the body of a pretty teenage girl walking by . . . grunts when he encounters two teenagers young enough to be his daughters . . . mutters, 'check out the hot blonde' to his buddy; the hot blonde is not yet 16."[27]

Some girls attempt to take control of their bodies by shrinking them until the self seems to disappear.

Prevention of eating disorders and dysfunctional eating needs to begin by dealing with the sexual harassment that goes on against young girls at the time when their bodies begin developing.

"I think if the women's movement has failed young girls in this country, which it clearly has, then they need a girls' movement,"

Levine says.[28]

Women must speak out forcefully about the dangers of the obsession with thinness, says Kilbourne. "This is not a trivial issue; it cuts to the very heart of women's energy, power and self-esteem. This is a major public health problem, one that endangers the lives of young girls and women."

Sexual harassment

"We believe sexual harassment is so pervasive that it is an integral part of 'normal' female development . . .

"In our work with young women, we have heard countless accounts of this contempt being expressed by their male peers: the girls who do not want to walk down a certain hallway in their high school because they are afraid of being publicly rated on a scale of one to ten; the girls who are subjected to barking, grunting and mooing calls and labels of 'dogs, cows or pigs' when they pass by groups of male students; those who are teased about not measuring up to buxom, bikini-clad (models); and the girls who are grabbed, pinched, groped and fondled as they try to make their way through the school corridors."

"Harassing words do not slide harmlessly away as the taunting sounds dissipate . . . They are slowly absorbed into the child's identity and developing sense of self, becoming an essential part of whom she sees herself to be. Harassment involves the use of words as weapons to inflict pain and assert power. Harassing words are meant to instill fear, heighten bodily discomfort, and diminish the sense of self."

JUNE LARKIN, CARLA RICE AND VANESSA RUSSELL
SLIPPING THROUGH THE CRACKS: SEXUAL HARASSMENT
EATING DISORDERS 1996;4:1:5-26

CHAPTER 3

Dysfunctional eating
disrupts normal life

■

Dysfunctional eating is a new term to describe the various kinds of inappropriate, abnormal, or problem eating behaviors which disrupt normal life, but not so severely as to be classified clinical eating disorders.

You may recognize the eating patterns. The junior high girl who skips breakfast and lunch, has a candy bar and Diet Coke after school, finds a way to skip the evening meal with her family — and then goes on an eating binge in the evening. The 4th grader who eats only a small amount of each food on her plate, never feeling really satisfied, because she's afraid of getting fat. The wrestler who fasts for two days before his match, to make weight, then eats nonstop another two days. The high school student who refuses meat, eggs, milk or any foods she thinks could make her "fat."

This kind of eating hasn't been investigated in much detail. Yet concerned leaders have been writing about various aspects of it for more than a decade. Children are growing up with skewed attitudes toward food, eating and weight because of fear of fat. They are turning away from normal eating and mealtimes with their families to restrained and chaotic eating.

Yet, dieting — a form of dysfunctional eating — starts as young as age nine, and by age 11 is so common that some researchers have called it the norm.

A growing number of studies document this disturbing trend. More than half of 14-year-old girls in a study of 1,000 suburban Chicago girls had already been on at least one weight loss diet.[1] Similarly, 30 to 46 percent of nine-year-old girls and 46 to 81 percent of 10-year-old girls in a California study had disordered eating, restricting their food due to fear of fat.[2]

If dysfunctional eating is becoming so prevalent, we need to know more about it. It's time to take a closer look. What is abnormal, problem eating? What are its effects? How can it be measured?

What is dysfunctional eating?

Dysfunctional eating is eating which is separated or disjoined from its normal function and normal internal controls.

Normal eating nourishes the body for health, energy and strength, enhancing feelings of well-being and resulting in "feeling good." Dysfunctional eating is often focused on eating for thinness, body shaping, or using food for comfort or emotional reasons. After eating, it is common to feel guilty, ashamed, uncomfortably full, to regret or berate oneself for having eating or, if unsatisfied, to feel ravenously hungry and fear or anticipate an onrushing eating binge.

Normal eating is controlled by an internal system that regulates the balance of food intake with expenditure, through hunger, appetite and satiety signals, so that a person eats when hungry and stops when full and satisfied. Normal eating is flexible and includes eating for pleasure and social reasons. In normal eating a person usually follows regular habits, such as eating three meals and snacks to satisfy hunger.

This is the way babies, small children and even animals eat. But it appears that by age 11 most girls are no longer eating this way, at least not on an everyday basis.

Dysfunctional eating exists on a continuum or range between normal eating and eating disorders *(see charts on pages 48-49)*. It may be of mild, moderate or severe intensity. Individuals may move back and forth across the continuum, returning to normal eating after unsuccessful bouts of dieting, or restricting so severely they develop debilitating eating disorders from which they cannot recover alone.

Dysfunctional eating includes the various kinds of eating patterns which have been called restrained eating, disordered eating, emotional eating, and chronic dieting syndrome. Its broader focus provides a framework for concerns and theory which have been nebulous and incompletely defined.

In contrast to normal eating, dysfunctional eating most often serves functions other than nourishment, such as to shape the body, improve body image, to seek comfort or pleasure, to numb pain or unhappy memory, to relieve stress, anxiety, anger, loneliness or boredom.

Dysfunctional eating is regulated by inappropriate external and internal controls, such as "will power," a planned diet, calories or fat grams, or emotional or sensory cues (seeing or smelling food). Though often the internal function is to relieve stress, it does not do this well. Instead of relieving pain, eating often makes the situation worse, or relief may be fleeting, followed by remorse.

Studies suggest that dysfunctional eating is extremely prevalent, especially among girls and women. It appears to be increasing and striking at younger ages as cultural pressures to be thin continue to increase. It may include at times as many as the 50 to 80 percent of girls and women in the U.S., age 11 and up, who report they are trying to lose weight. Increasingly, it includes teenage boys and men, who are responding to new advertising pressures to reshape their bodies.

Dysfunctional eating is unlikely for infants, small children and others who don't diet or have not learned to interfere with the normal eating process.

It includes variations of chaotic eating, as well as both persistent undereating and overeating. There are at least three general patterns: chaotic or irregular eating, consistent undereating, and consistent overeating of much more than the body wants or needs.

■ **Chaotic or irregular eating.** Many girls and young women, and some males, eat in chaotic or irregular ways: fasting, dieting, skipping meals, snacking often, restricting their eating at times, bingeing at others. They may have a fear of fat, body dissatisfaction, and a

Dysfunctional eating: a description

Contrasted and compared with normal eating and eating disorders

	Normal eating	Dysfunctional eating	Eating disorders
Eating pattern	Regular eating habits and patterns. Typical pattern in U.S. is to eat three regular meals and snacks to satisfy hunger.	Irregular, chaotic eating — often overeat or undereat, skip meals, fast, binge, diet. Or usual pattern is of overeating or undereating much more or much less than body wants or needs.	Patterns typical of anorexia nervosa, bulimia nervosa, binge eating disorder, other eating disorders.
Function, purpose of eating	Eat for nourishment, health, energy. Also for pleasure and social reasons. Eating enhances feelings of well-being, makes one "feel good."	Eating often for reasons other than nourishment: to shape body, improve body image, seek comfort or pleasure, numb pain, relieve stress, anxiety, anger, loneliness or boredom. May feel uncomfortable after eating, or have feelings of remorse, guilt, shame.	Eating almost entirely for purposes other than nourishment or energy, as for body shaping, to numb pain, relieve stress.
Use of hunger, appetite and satiety to regulate eating	Eating regulated by internal signals of hunger, appetite and satiety. Eat when hungry, stop when full and satisfied; usually hungry at mealtime.	Eating often separated from normal controls of hunger, appetite and satiety. May be regulated by "will power," a planned diet, calories or fat grams, emotional or sensory cues, such as sight or smell of food.	Eating regulated predominantly by external and internal controls other than hunger and satiety.
Prevalence	Infants, small children, persons who don't diet or interfere with normal eating. At this time, higher rates among males, fewer among females.	Chaotic eating and undereating affect many girls and women in U.S., perhaps at times as many as the 50 to 80% age 11 and over who say they are trying to lose weight; also increasing numbers of boys and men. Consistent overeating may occur for both genders.	Estimated prevalence is 10% of high school and college students; 90-95% female, 5-10% male.

Reprinted from *Afraid to Eat*, by Frances M. Berg. Copyright 1997. All rights reserved. Publisher's written permission required for reproduction. Published by Healthy Weight Journal, 402 South 14th Street, Hettinger, ND 58639 (701-567-2646; Fax 701-567-2602).

Dysfunctional eating: effects and relationships

	Normal eating	Dysfunctional eating			Eating disorders
		mild	*moderate*	*severe*	
Physical	Promotes health, energy, strength, and the healthy growth and development of children and youth.	May typically feel tired, apathetic, lacking in energy, chilled. Increased risk of stunted growth and reduced brain development with undernutrition. Decreased bone development or bone demineralization and higher risk of fractures. Delayed pubery, decrease in sexual interest.			Physical effects may be severe. Mortality reportedly as high as 18% for anorexia nervosa and bulimia nervosa.
	WEIGHT: Normal weight for the individual, expressing genetic and environmental factors. Any weight within wide range; usually stable.	WEIGHT: Any weight within wide range depending on genetic potential. Eating pattern may cause weight to decrease, cycle up and down, remain stable, or increase.			WEIGHT: Any weight within wide range, depending on genetic potential and the disorder and its expression.
Mental focus	Promotes clear thinking, ability to concentrate.	Risk of decreased mental alertness and ability to concentrate, narrowing of interests, loss of ambition, and a turning inward.			Diminished capacity to think, memory loss, extreme narrowing of interests.
	FOOD THOUGHTS: low key, usually at mealtime. For women, 10-15% of time awake may be spent thinking of food, hunger, weight.	FOOD THOUGHTS: Increased preoccupation with food. Thoughts often focused on eating, weight, planning when and what to eat, counting calories or fat grams. Thoughts of food, hunger, weight may occupy 20-65% of time.			FOOD THOUGHTS: Thoughts focused most of time on food, hunger, weight. For untreated anorexia about 90-110%, bulimia 70-90% of time awake (extra 10% includes dreaming).
Emotional	Promotes mood stability.	Potentially greater mood instability — highs and lows. May be easily upset, irritable, anxious, have lowered self-esteem. Increasing preoccupation and concern with body image. Increased risk of eating disorders.			Greater risk of mood instability and functional depression.
Social	Social integration; promotes healthy relationships with family, peers and community.	Less social integration, more risk of feeling isolated, self-absorbed and self-focused, stigmatized, disconnected from society, lonely. May have less interest in values of generosity, sharing, volunteer activities; less sense of community.			Social withdrawal, isolated from family and friends, avoidance of and by peers, alienation, often eating alone; worsening family relations.

Reprinted from *Afraid to Eat*, by Frances M. Berg. Copyright 1997. All rights reserved. Publisher's written permission required for reproduction. Published by Healthy Weight Journal, 402 South 14th Street, Hettinger, ND 58639 (701-567-2646; Fax 701-567-2602).

strong desire to change their bodies in ways they perceive as being more socially desirable.

■ **Undereating.** Many girls and young women, and some males, eat less food on a daily basis than meets their daily needs and requirements for healthy growth and development. They may be "dieting successes," and may develop anorexic eating patterns, even though they do not meet the clinical criteria of anorexia nervosa. Today these are frequent reports: teenage girls with daily intakes consisting of only lettuce, or an apple or bagel, or perhaps "half a raisin"; a college sorority in which members pay a penalty if they eat any fat at all; a dancing troupe in which fat may be eaten but not swallowed. These young women are able to successfully restrict their eating so that they maintain a thin or extremely thin body which is lower than expected, given their genetic and environmental heritage. Yet, despite their success, they may be dissatisfied with their body shape and size. Other reasons for undereating may be because of depression, alcoholism, or other mental or physical factors.

■ **Overeating.** Many children and youth may eat more food on a daily basis than their bodies want or need, eating past satiety, and well above growth needs. They may overeat from emotional or stress-related reasons, such as for comfort, to relieve stress or boredom, to deal with anger or resentment. Or they may overeat from family or peer group habits of eating large amounts of food, or eating more because plenty of good tasting foods are readily available. Body size is not to be taken as an indicator of this type of dysfunctional eating. It cannot be assumed that large persons are eating abnormally, or past the point of satiety. In the U.S. today, studies suggest that overeating is being encouraged. People are eating out more, and they favor fast food chains and restaurants where they perceive they are getting more for their money. In response, studies show restaurants are offering larger servings and larger meals. Conditions such as Prader-Willi syndrome, which involves a disruption of hunger, appetite and satiety regulation, may or may not fit into this category.

The above patterns of dysfunctional eating can also include youngsters who undereat, overeat, or eat erratically because of involuntary factors such as depression, disease or insufficient food.

Physical effects

The person with dysfunctional eating may often feel tired and lacking in energy, especially when undernourished. There is risk of stunted growth and reduced brain development in children and teens, according to poverty studies worldwide. Bone development may be decreased for youth; for young women increased bone demineralization may occur, leading to bone fractures. Puberty may be delayed and sexual interest decreased.

Dysfunctional eating affects weight, yet in its various forms it is associated with a wide range of weights as genetic potential interacts with environmental lifestyle factors. Associated with chaotic eating and dieting, weight often cycles up and down in "yo-yo" fashion. Consistent undereating can be expected to result in a stable weight lower than normal for that person. Overeating will likely result in a higher weight than might be normal for that individual, perhaps increasing year by year.

Mental focus

One of the most dramatic effects of dysfunctional eating may be its impact on the thinking process.

As dysfunctional eating becomes more severe, the individual often loses mental focus, mental alertness and the ability to concentrate. Her interests may narrow, turning inward, and she loses ambition. As interest in food heightens she tends to lose interest in school work, career, family and friends, and pulls back from social activities. This may be the girl primarily occupied with boyfriends who wants to marry right out of high school. Anorectic girls tend to be popular with boys, says Mary Pipher, they are very feminine, thin, passive and eager to please.

This increase in food preoccupation is clear in the wartime Minnesota Human Starvation study, and more recently has been researched by Dan Reiff, MPH, RD, and Kim Lampson Reiff, PhD, a husband-wife eating disorder team in Mercer Island, Wash.[3]

In their book, *Eating Disorders: Nutrition Therapy in the Recovery Process,* the Reiffs provide a food preoccupation scale. Individuals are asked to indicate total conscious time spent thinking about food, weight and hunger at three times in their lives (currently, at its highest, and at its lowest) and to give their age and weight for each. This includes time spent in shopping, preparing food, eating, thinking

---

Eating Attitudes Test

(EAT) Sample questions

Choose the answer that best applies:
Always - Very often - Often - Sometimes - Rarely - Never

1. I am scared about being overweight.

2. I stay away from eating when I am hungry.

3. I think about food a lot of the time.

4. I have gone on eating binges where I feel that I might not be able to stop.

5. I cut my food into small pieces.

6. I am aware of the calorie content in foods I eat.

7. I feel guilty after eating.

8. I vomit after I have eaten.

9. I think about burning up calories when I exercise.

10. I stay away from foods with sugar [or fat] in them.

11. I feel that others pressure me to eat.

12. I like my stomach to be empty.[1]

From Garner and Garfinkel's Eating Attitudes Test
Children's version, by Maloney, et. al.

about eating or food cravings, purging, weighing, reading diet books, suppressing feelings of hunger, using strategies such as smoking or chewing gum to distract from hunger, and thinking about or discussing weight.

The researchers tested more than 500 eating disordered patients on this scale. They found that for untreated anorexia nervosa patients, 90 to 110 percent of waking time is spent thinking about food, weight and hunger. The extra 10 percent comes from dreams of food or weight, or having their sleep disturbed by hunger. Bulimic patients report about 70 to 90 percent.

From the testing he has done, Dan Reiff suggests that for women with normal eating, who are buying and preparing food for the family, the amount of time spent thinking about food, weight and hunger may be about 10 to 15 percent of waking time. In dysfunctional eating, this may occupy about 20 to 65 percent of waking hours, he reports.

In his studies, preoccupation with food is directly related to body weight and the degree and duration of semi-starvation.

In the Keys' Minnesota study, it appeared to be most closely related to the drop in body weight, as the men consumed a fairly adequate diet of 1,500 to 1,700 calories for six months, but lost one-fourth of their weight.

Eating disorder risk

A major concern with the current high prevalence of dysfunctional eating is whether it will lead to increased rates of eating disorders. Undoubtedly, many girls and young women who begin by dieting and restricting food move on to clinical eating disorders.

A recent review reports that several one to two year longitudinal studies have shown that up to 35 percent of normal dieters progress to pathological dieting, and of pathological dieters, 20 to 25 percent progress to partial or full syndrome disorders.

The report also says that 15 to 45 percent of those with partial syndrome progress to full syndrome eating disorders within one to four years.[4]

Emotional changes

Dysfunctional eating can have severe emotional effects. The individual may become moody, easily upset, irritable, anxious, apathetic, increasingly concerned about body image. She is often self-absorbed and self-focused. Self-esteem may be low, or focused on appearance.

The girl with dysfunctional eating may isolate herself socially, feeling lonely, alienated, and disconnected from society. She may focus less than others on the values of generosity, sharing, caring, and participate less in volunteer and community activities.

Survival traits

Can some of these abnormal eating effects be explained as survival traits that kept our ancestors alive? I believe they can, particularly those factors related to undernutrition.

Early humans must have frequently feasted weeks on the carcass of a mammoth or beached whale, then gone into a period of famine during which they were semi-starved for months or even the proverbial seven years. In deprivation, their bodies would have shut down to conserve fuel, not just with slowed heart rate and metabolism, but in every activity. Growth stopped or was severely stunted. Nearly all fat consumed was routed to storage to replace what was lost, instead of being used normally. Sexual activity and fertility shut down; as starvation progressed it was more critical to care for the young than to procreate. Ultimately, even children were abandoned, as Colin Turnbull reports so vividly in *The Mountain People*.

At the same time, starvation causes high stress. There is no peace for starving people. They crave food and focus all attention on this overriding need. A useful survival trait, this kept our ancestors out hunting food despite weakness or danger, instead of lying listless in the cave, awaiting death.

When food was plentiful, the once-starved people ate more and more often. Their natural efficiency increased to ward off the expected effects of the next famine. Without this internal regulation, the human race could hardly have survived. But this ancient legacy haunts the dysfunctional eater today.

Cultural pressures encourage dysfunction

American culture today encourages these kinds of dysfunctional, disturbed and disruptive eating patterns. Youngsters are being coaxed to overeat and at the same time, urged to restrict their eating. They are persuaded to override their internal control systems and to take on the responsibility of shaping their bodies according to the narrow ideals prescribed by society.

Normal eating is not being encouraged.

We have plenty of inexpensive, good-tasting foods, easily available. And a culture of eating for pleasure has developed, molded by the advertising millions are spent each year to promote it. Restaurants report that customers are expecting larger portion sizes and they are responding with bigger servings and more abundant buffets.

A recent study reported in *Restaurants USA* found customers expected larger quantities of food in 1993 than in 1991, and that people think of large servings as getting better value for their money when they eat out.[5]

A subscriber in London recently sent me a newspaper story titled "Portions out of all proportion" that decry America's "elephantine cuisine." It compares the size of hot dogs (350 calories in the U.S., 150 in Britain), cookies (493 vs 65), ice cream cone (625 vs 160), muffin (705 vs 158), nachos (1,650 vs 569), and a meal of steak and fries (2,060 vs 730).

Until recently, our large muffins were called "jumbo muffins," the article notes; now they are simply "muffins."

The Cheesecake Factory heaps food "practically a foot high on its plates and proudly serves up a 12 ounce burger. As for the cheesecake, each slice has about 700 calories. It claims it tried to serve lower-calorie slices but nobody wanted them."

And I detect a bit of a British sniff which, yes, we deserve: "Europeans are a lot more quality conscious . . . Americans just want value for their money, and base value on size."

At the same time we are being encouraged to eat more, dieting and thinness are even more heavily promoted. Thinness is a potent advertising theme being used to create body dissatisfaction and sell products of all kinds, from diet pills to fashions and cigarettes. The health community has joined with advertisers and the media in fervently promoting these thin ideals and the need for children, as well as adults, to reshape their bodies in so-called "healthier" ways.

Both extremes appeal to external regulation of eating and to eating for purposes other than to nourish the body for its optimal health and performance. They ignore the fact that our bodies are wonderfully designed to maintain their own balance through internal regulating systems.

Moreover, there is an intense fear of food in the U.S. today. People are confused and worried about the foods they eat.

"I've never known so many people to be so worried about what they eat, or so many who think of the dinner table as a trap that's killing them," says Julia Child, the noted chef and author. Child is involved in the "Resetting the American Table" project by nutritionists, chefs, educators and product developers, which aims to help people rediscover the joys of eating while moving toward a healthier diet.

The project confronts the damaging effect of "our largely single-focused messages, especially messages urging restriction of food choices or based on fear of disease."[6]

It promotes eating good food with friends and family as a pleasurable and healthful experience.

How eating patterns develop

The origins of dysfunctional eating and its development are not well understood. The effects of a bout of restrained eating may perpetuate more disturbed eating, say Linda Smolak and Michael Levine, eating disorder specialists. This may even begin, not as a desire for thinness, but simply through following the examples or encouragement of parents or peers. When children begin dieting early, they may gradually develop intensified disrupted eating patterns that lead to fully-developed eating disorders.

"Such disregulated eating may take the form of more stringent and frequent dieting, as well as binge eating. Thus, the children who are already dieting during elementary school may be at risk for developing eating disorders because of the physiological and psychological effects of caloric restriction and weight loss failures."

Another pathway to fully-developed eating disorders may be the cultural pressures to be thin.

"Girls who put enough stake in the importance of thinness may find it necessary to go to extremes in order to attain the desired look, resulting in body dissatisfaction, dieting and exercising for weight control and, perhaps, eating disorders," say Smolak and Levine.

Their research indicates that in grades one to five, a subgroup of girls believes that "thinness is important in determining whether a girl is pretty."[7]

Dysfunctional eating may not be so very different from clinical eating disorders. For some it's just a matter of degree. It's no longer possible to dismiss patients with severe eating disorders as uniquely pathological, as was often done in the past, say eating disorder specialists.

They may simply be expressing what many other girls and women across the eating spectrum are feeling.[8] Chronic dieters and those who fear fat experience the same kinds of mental and physical harm to the degree that they practice self-starvation, abuse of diet pills, purging and similar behaviors.

Normal eating

Unlike these types of disruptive eating, normal eating is positive and flexible and depends on internal cues for regulation. Ellyn Satter, RD, an eating disorder specialist and international specialist on childhood feeding has given us an excellent definition of normal eating in her book, *How to Get Your Kid to Eat . . . But Not Too Much.*

"Normal eating is being able to eat when you are hungry and continue eating until you are satisfied. It is being able to choose food you like and eat it and truly get enough of it — not just stop eating because you think you should. Normal eating is being able to use some moderate constraint in your food selection to get the right food, but not being so restrictive that you miss out on pleasurable foods.

"Normal eating is giving yourself permission to eat sometimes because you are happy, sad or bored, or just because it feels good. Normal eating is three meals a day, most of the time, but it can also be choosing to munch along . . . Normal eating is trusting your body to make up for your mistakes in eating.

"In short, normal eating is flexible. It varies in response to your emotions, your schedule, your hunger, and your proximity to food."

Family attitudes

Family attitudes about weight can set the stage for developing disordered eating.

These attitudes may be evident in constant family dieting, and using restriction, compulsive eating, overeating or excessive exercising to control anxiety, as well as making disparaging comments about one's own body, and being obsessed with appearance — especially body image and weight, according to Dan Reiff and Kathleen Kim Lampson Reiff, Mercer Island, Wash., authors of *Eating Disorders.*[9]

The Reiffs point out that a father or mother talking with disrespect or strong disapproval about the body shape or weight of the other parent who is overweight teaches the child to fear such responses from her parents, boyfriends or spouse regarding her body. Or parents and siblings making critical remarks about other people who are overweight may convince the child that at all costs she must never become overweight or she too will be unacceptable.

The uneasy relationships that mothers have with food and with their bodies, are mirrored in their daughters at very young ages. Satter advises parents to model normal eating. "If you diet constantly . . . If your eating is fragile and chaotic and fraught with anxiety, (your child's) chances are increased of learning to eat in much the same way."

Satter says parents should purchase, prepare and serve food, but allow the child to choose what and how much he or she will eat. Unfortunately this natural division of responsibility is often violated by parents with rigid or restricting eating styles of their own, who try to take over their children's eating, she reports. This sets the stage for disruptive and disturbed eating styles.

It's a hard point to get across to people, she says, but "Even the fat child is entitled to regulate the amount of food he eats."

Putting a child on a diet

Disruption of normal eating may occur when parents fear a child is gaining too much weight, and they begin to restrict his or her food. Deprivation diets can stimulate changes that foster disordered eating and weight gain, says Laurel Mellin, RD, MA, University of California, San Francisco. She reports that obese youngsters are at greater risk for developing disordered eating than normal-weight youth.[10]

Never put a child on a diet, Satter advises. "Diets are not an option. Restricting food intake, even in indirect ways, profoundly distorts developmental needs of children and adolescents."

She says it's time to define problems of childhood obesity in ways they can be solved, rather than continuing to set patients up for failure by putting them on weight loss diets. "In my view, no person has the right to impose starvation on another, even if that other person is your child. Withholding food profoundly interferes with a child's autonomy, and you will both pay the price."

Research needed

The adverse factors associated with dysfunctional eating and its high prevalence make further study imperative. The concept covers a complexity of issues. Indeed, it is amazing how powerful the associations reveal themselves when we see the big picture.

Much research is needed in these areas.

How can we identify and measure the various patterns of dysfunctional eating? What causes the related adverse effects: is it abnormal eating habits, insufficient calories, iron or other nutrient deficiencies, weight loss, depleted fat cells, or psychological factors?

If dysfunctional eating is unhealthy, as it appears to be, how can it be prevented? How can normal eating be restored for children and adult women? Normal eating itself needs study. What is normal eating and does it have its own range of patterns? How can it be measured?

A note of caution: The case made here for normal eating is not meant to imply that nutrition is the primary factor in good mental and physical health, but rather, that each person has a baseline of adequate nutrition, (and perhaps an upper level, as well), and when this is disrupted there may severe disruption of normal life and a diminishing of mind, body and spirit.

Only when food supply is stable can people eat and live normally, as we interpret this today. With adequate nutrition and regular eating habits, they can focus on developing their full potential through a wide range of interests. They can afford the luxury of being generous, sharing, caring, and reaching out to others.

Research basis

The concepts of dysfunctional eating I've brought together are defined here for the first time, yet they are based on the insight and research of numerous leaders in the fields of obesity, eating disorders and size acceptance. Much of it is contained in our 1995 special report, *Health Risks of Weight Loss*.

Concerned leaders have been writing about this for more than a decade.

Still most striking to me are the classic Toronto milkshake studies of the early 1980s that showed that the more milkshakes restrained eaters drank before supper, the more food they ate. And I've been moved by the wartime Minnesota studies of men who opposed war but went on an austere six-month diet to help starving people in war-torn countries, and even more by Turnbull's terrible revelations in *The Mountain People* of what really happens to society and family life during starvation. More recently, I've been alarmed to learn how much of their lives people who eat abnormally devote to thinking about food and self, and how little to others.

And I'm reminded that everywhere in our country, today and every day, women and young girls are doing this to themselves and having it done to them by health professionals and con artists, as the screws tighten on them to become thinner and ever thinner.

In the 11 years I've been publishing *Healthy Weight Journal*, I've read nearly every scrap of research and insight on this topic (my library on weight and eating research, part of which lies in piles on my office floor, has been called the most extensive in the world, and I believe it may be — what library can afford the wonderful review books, journals and reports that arrive here daily?).

What I'm seeing is an increase in dysfunctional eating, its engulfing of ever younger children, and national increases in related adverse effects, while many in the health and medical communities (with their shepherds the diet companies) continue to increase pressures on Americans to lose weight.

Changing all this cannot be easy, but perhaps bringing it together into this kind of framework will help. If women can learn how dieting disrupts normal life, will they be so quick to discard life's richness for the preoccupation of watching a few pounds come and go? Perhaps they will awaken with a start, restore normal eating in their homes, reach out with love and caring, and become — with their children — whole again in mind, body and spirit.

This is my hope.

*Dieters are people who get up in the
morning and the first thing they say is:
"Mirror, mirror, on the dresser —
do I look a little lesser?"*

ROBERT ORBEN
WALL STREET JOURNAL

CHAPTER 4

Eating disorders
shatter young lives

■

As American adults continue to obsess about weight and diet, it is hardly surprising that eating disorders among their children have risen to crisis levels.

Prevalence has been difficult to determine because of the extremes sufferers take to hide their disorder and public health apathy in compiling statistics. The best estimate is that about one in 10 teenagers and college students wrestle with eating disorders — severe disturbances in eating behavior usually driven by a fear of being fat.

While overweight may carry health risks over a lifetime, some eating disorders, like anorexia nervosa, can be deadly and take but a few years to kill. An estimated 10 percent to 15 percent of anorexia nervosa patients die of their illness. Some say the mortality is as high as 18 percent.[1]

Those who survive find the road to recovery difficult. While in the grip of the disorder, health, jobs, school and relationships all suffer — and rebuilding can be a serious, and sometimes insurmountable, challenge. For many there are irreversible physical and mental changes due to malnutrition and purging. Less than half, about 44 percent, have overall good recovery; about 31 percent are intermediate, and 25 percent have a poor outcome.

Eating disorders take inordinate amounts of time and concentration — time taken from other relationships and normal activities. They can be associated with alcohol and/or drug abuse, which can increase the medical and mental complications. Sufferers lose energy, irritate easily, find themselves lonely and driven to keep their disorder a secret.

Common symptoms include fatigue, lethargy, weakness, impaired concentration, nonfocal abdominal pain, dizziness, faintness, sore muscles, chills, cold sweats frequent sore throats, diarrhea and constipation, according to Allan Kaplan and Paul Garfinkel in Medical issues and the Eating Disorders.

"I have many regrets. I lost a number of friends, hurt a lot of people I care about," laments one young woman who recovered from anorexia nervosa and bulimia nervosa. "My memories of the last 16 years are spotty and dim. In fact, there have been many major events, such as my sister's wedding, that I have no recollection of. Eighty to 90 percent of my time was spent in [eating] behaviors. My behaviors overtook my life and I essentially lost 16 years of living — years that I can't have back."[2]

With eating disorders come feelings of loss of control, of helplessness. There is alienation from family.

The father of a child with an eating disorder said, "She has withdrawn into her own world. She's lonely and is missing out on all the fun and exciting things during her teenage years . . . I have cried many times over this."[3]

Families of youth with eating disorders are in a difficult situation. They see the child behaving in a destructive way and may feel helpless and frustrated over what to do. They may try to gain control over what and how much the teenager chooses to eat. Some police washrooms, or go through drawers for diet pills or laxatives. Most parents struggle with both the eating behavior and concerns over injury to their growth and development. The eating disorder can take over most aspects of family life.

Many specialists in the field are convinced that the current high rates of eating disorders in the U.S. are the inevitable result of 60 to

80 million adults dieting, losing weight, rebounding, and learning to be chronic dieters. The majority of these are women.[4]

Prevalence

Eating disorders affect an estimated 7 percent of community populations and 10 percent of student populations, according to most estimates. These are not solid statistics based on national figures, however, and many experts suggest the figures are actually much higher. There is some debate on whether prevalence of severe eating disorders has increased during the last decade.

Most of the eating disorder specialists I network with and many writers in the field are saying not only that prevalence has increased considerably, but that it has increased greatly for males, and is striking both girls and boys at younger ages.

About 9,000 people are hospitalized annually in the U.S. for the treatment of eating disorders, according to Robin Sesan, PhD, director of the Brandywine Psychotherapy Center Wilmington, Del.[5]

Widely regarded as a modern problem, eating disorders have been known for centuries. For some time it was thought eating disorders are more common in middle and upper socioeconomic levels, but there is increasing recognition that they affect people of all economic levels, genders and ethnicities.[6]

Eating disorders usually consist of two sets of disturbances: First, those related to food and weight, and second, those concerning relationships with oneself and others. They are extremely complex, rising out of both emotional problems and eating disturbances, and within a culture that puts great emphasis on thinness and appearance. Some problems may be rooted in families that are overly controlling or disengaged, or who are having problems they are unable to acknowledge or deal with openly. Puberty may be a critical time.

Often sexual abuse or trauma will be an initiating event. Some specialists see eating disorders as survival strategies developed in response to harassment, racism, homophobia, abuse of power, poverty, or emotional, physical or sexual abuse.

The term "eating disorder" is somewhat misleading because it implies the main problem is eating, to be solved by learning to eat normally again. Given the complex behavioral and psychological components of eating disorders, it isn't that simple.

Yet, dieting itself is increasingly being regarded as an important risk factor in developing eating disorders.

Dieting disorders

"Eating disorders should be called dieting disorders, because it is the dieting process and not eating that causes the initiation of both anorexia nervosa and bulimia nervosa," says Joe McVoy, PhD, an eating disorder specialist in Radford, Va.

McVoy says the term "eating disorder" seems to indicate something is wrong with the eating process, whereas what happens is a conscious choice to restrict one's food intake or diet, which leads to starvation and ultimately the disorder.

"Onset of an eating disorder typically follows a period of restrictive dieting; however, only a minority of people who diet develop eating disorders," says the American Dietetic Association in its position paper on eating disorders.[7]

A study of 15-year-old girls in London linked dieting to the development of eating disorders. Those initially dieting were significantly more likely than nondieters to develop an eating disorder within one year. Only 21 percent of the girls were dieting at the beginning of the study, but they were eight times more likely to develop an eating disorder later.[8]

The American Dietetic Association warns against promoting weight loss to persons with binge eating disorder or other eating disorders, as it can be very detrimental to their physical and mental health.

Often large youngsters with these disorders may be referred to the dietitian for help in losing weight. The ADA position paper recommends counseling on body image issues and how to stop the pursuit of thinness. It may be healthier to suggest that young people accept themselves at or near their present weight, stop binge eating and learn how to prevent future weight gain.

Anorexia nervosa

"When I first started to eat strangely, all I would eat were sweets, and that wasn't any good. Then I got into just eating salads, just lettuce and diet pop, and that wasn't any good. Then I got into pretty much not eating at all, and that wasn't any good," said a former anorexic patient quoted in Eating Disorders.[9]

Anorexia nervosa affects about 1 in 500 adolescents (0.2 percent), 90 to 95 percent of them female, according to the National Eating Disorders Organization.4 Some studies find rates as high as 1 in 100 girls between ages 12 and 18 (1 percent). Follow-up studies show death rates as high as 18 percent for anorexia nervosa and bulimia nervosa, report Dan Reiff and Kathleen Kim Lampson Reiff.[10]

The disorder has had some high-profile victims. Singer Karen Carpenter. Gymnast Christy Heinrich.

Actress Tracey Gold, of the ABC sitcom "Growing Pains," was only 12 when her pediatrician first diagnosed her anorexia. Four months of psychotherapy seemed to get the problem under control and she gained weight, up to 133 pounds by the time she turned 19 in 1988. It was too much, she thought. To lose weight her endocrinologist put her on a 500-calorie-a-day-diet and in two months she had dropped to her goal of 113. But during the next three years her weight kept dropping, until in January 1992 at 80 pounds she was hospitalized and had to fight to save her life. Two years later, "now rosy-skinned" and feeling "healthy enough to know I don't want to lose any more," she still panicked at the thought of reaching 100 pounds, and had brought her weight only up to 92 pounds.[11]

In anorexia nervosa, by definition the individual is more than 15 percent under expected weight, fears gaining weight, is preoccupied with food, has abnormal eating habits, and has amenorrhea, or if male, a decrease in sexual drive or interest. There are two types: one simply restricts food, the other restricts food and either purges regularly, or binges and purges both, according to the *APA Diagnostic and Statistical Manual.*

Changes occur in behavior, perception, thinking, mood and social interaction. A sense of heightened control and control over food seems important to the person with anorexia. Pleasure and enjoyment during

Diagnostic criteria

Anorexia nervosa

Patients with anorexia nervosa refuse to maintain weight at or above what is minimally normal for age and height (less than 85% of expected weight), and have an intense fear of weight gain or becoming fat. They have disturbance in body image, causing undue influence on self-esteem. If female, they have amenorrhea, defined as the absence of at least three consecutive menstrual cycles.

Two types are:

- **Restricting type**: severely restrict food without regularly binge eating or purging.
- **Binge eating/purging type:** with binge eating or purging (induced vomiting or misuse of laxatives, diuretics or enemas).

Bulimia nervosa

In bulimia nervosa the individual has recurrent episodes of binge eating. An episode includes eating, in a discrete period of time, an amount of food larger than most people would eat, and a sense of lack of control over what or how much one is eating during the episode. It includes recurrent inappropriate compensatory behavior to prevent weight gain, such as induced vomiting, misuse of laxatives, diuretics, enemas, or other medications; fasting; or excessive exercise. Both binge eating and the compensatory behavior occur at least twice a week for three months, on average. One's self-evaluation is unduly influenced by body shape and weight. (The disturbance does not occur exclusively during episodes of anorexia nervosa.)

Two types are:

- **Purging type:** uses regular purging behavior (induced vomiting or misuse of laxatives, diuretics or enemas).
- **Nonpurging type:** uses other inappropriate compensatory behaviors, such as fasting or excessive exercise, but does not regularly engage in purging.[1]

From Diagnostic criteria for eating disorders. Diagnostic and Statistical Manual, Fourth Edition, 1994. American Psychiatric Association, Washington, DC.

eating are replaced by guilt, anxiety and ambivalence. Mood tends to be depressed, irritable, anxious and unstable often leading to increased social isolation. Compulsive exercising may be a part of the disorder.

Symptoms are usually evident: emaciated appearance, dry skin, sometimes yellowish, fine body hair, brittle hair and nails, body temperature below 96.6, pulse rate usually below 60 beats per minute, subnormal blood pressure, and sometimes edema, say Kaplan and Garfinkel.

Initially, these are similar to symptoms associated with a restrictive diet: light-headedness, apathy, irritability, and decrease in energy. Then the consequences of prolonged semi-starvation begin to set in and the effects worsen. Duration of the disorder may range from a single episode to a lifelong illness.

Hospitalization may be required depending on body weight, the amount and rapidity of weight lost, severe metabolic disturbances, certain cardiac dysfunctions, syncope, psychomotor retardation, severe depression or suicide risk, severe bingeing and purging (with risk of aspiration), psychosis, family crisis, inability to perform activities of daily living, or lack of response to outpatient treatment programs. Most severely underweight patients, under 20 percent below average weight for height, and those who are psychologically unstable will require a residential setting.[12]

Families as well as patients will usually need psychotherapy.

Female athletes and dancers are at high risk for anorexia nervosa. As many as 13 to 22 percent of young women in selected groups of elite runners and dancers have the disorder. Two studies of female dancers cited by Jacqueline Berning and Suzanne Steen, authors of *Sports Nutrition for the 90's,* found between 5 and 22 percent had anorexia nervosa, with a higher incidence among young women competing in national rather than regional performances.[13]

Bulimia Nervosa

"I can't stop throwing up. I try, I really do. Yesterday, I promised myself I wouldn't do it anymore. I tried to keep myself busy. I cleaned house, played with the cat, prayed. . . But I don't want to gain weight. I can't do that! I never want to be fat again. I'll never

Eating disorder not otherwise specified

The third and largest eating disorder category is *Eating disorder not other wise specified*. Individuals in this category do not meet the definitions for either anorexia nervosa or bulimia nervosa.

Examples are:

- All criteria met for anorexia nervosa except amenorrhea.
- All criteria met for anorexia nervosa except, despite weight loss, current weight is in normal range.
- All criteria met for bulimia nervosa except frequency of binges is less than twice a week or for a duration of less than three months.
- An individual of normal body weight who regularly engages in inappropriate compensatory behavior (such as induced vomiting) after eating small amounts of food
- Repeatedly chewing and spitting out large amounts of food, without swallowing.
- Binge eating disorder.

Binge eating disorder

Binge eating disorder is a subtype under the category *Eating disorder not otherwise specified*. It is defined as recurrent episodes of binge eating, which includes eating, in a discrete period of time, an amount of food larger than most people would eat, and a sense of lack of control over eating it. The individual has marked distress regarding binge eating, and engages in binge eating on average, at least 2 days a week for 6 months. (The binge eating is not associated with the regular use of inappropriate compensatory behaviors and does not occur exclusively during the course of anorexia nervosa or bulimia nervosa.)

At least three of the following must be part of the binge episode:

- Eating much more rapidly than normal.
- Eating until uncomfortably full.
- Eating large amounts of food when not hungry.
- Eating alone because of embarrassment about how much is eaten.
- Feeling disgusted with oneself, depressed, or very guilty about eating.[1]

From Diagnostic criteria for eating disorders. Diagnostic and Statistical Manual, Fourth Edition, 1994. American Psychiatric Association, Washington, DC.

go back there. Nothing is worse than that pain. . .My joints even hurt. I feel so old. My hair looks horrible; and it keeps falling out. I find it all over the place. My mouth is so full of sores, it's gross! I can't even walk around the house standing straight any more. I'm in a daze. I can't focus. But I can't stop. I feel so trapped. Please help me..." said a patient from Lemon Grove, Calif., reported in *The Healthy Weigh.*[14]

Bulimia nervosa affects 1 to 3 percent of adolescents, according to the *Diagnostic and Statistical Manual,* 1994, American Psychiatric Association. A recent study of college freshmen found 4.5 percent of females and 0.4 percent of males had a history of bulimia nervosa, say the Reiffs.

The National Eating Disorder Information Centre in Canada reports somewhat higher figures for North America. These estimates are as follows: 1 percent to 3 percent of women in the population have anorexia nervosa, 3 percent to 5 percent have bulimia, and another 10 percent to 20 percent engage in some of the symptoms on an occasional basis. Both anorexia and bulimia can have severe physical and emotional effects, and in 10 to 20 percent of cases they can be fatal, warns the Centre.[15]

By definition, a person with bulimia nervosa goes on an eating binge at least twice a week, eating a very large amount of food within a discrete period and then tries to compensate for this either by purging or nonpurging behavior.

As the disorder progresses it develops into a complex lifestyle that is increasingly isolating from social relationships, with feelings of isolation, depressed mood and low self-esteem.

Vomiting is the most common form of purging. Some binge and purge many times a day. Patients with bulimia may be of normal weight and seem physically healthy — except for the telltale signs of vomiting behavior: finger calluses or lesions on the dominant hand from stimulating the gag reflex (especially in early stages when stimulation is needed to induce vomiting), "chipmunk" cheeks from stimulation of the salivary glands, erosion of enamel especially on the surface of the upper teeth next to the tongue.[16]

The consequences of the self-abusive purging behavior become increasingly obvious as the frequency and duration increase, and include hair loss, fatigue, insomnia, muscle weakness, edema, dizziness, sore throat, stomach pain or cramping, bloating, bad breath and bloodshot eyes. Cardiac arrhythmias affect 20 percent and require emergency treatment. Ipecac syrup abuse may lead to death through cardiomyopathy, myocarditis.

Up to one-third of anorexic individuals develop bulimia nervosa. Bulimia was only recognized in 1980 and listed by the American Psychiatric Association in its *Diagnostic and Statistical Manual.* In 1987 this was replaced by the term bulimia nervosa. It is unclear whether this was a hidden syndrome for many years, or if it is relatively new.

Bizarre behaviors

Many of the physical and mental abnormalities of eating disorders are known to chronic dieters and people who severely restrict their food intake.

The bizarre eating behaviors common to anorexia nervosa are typical of those described under other starvation conditions. In Ancel Keys' well-known Minnesota research studying the effects of famine in male volunteers who reduced their food intake by 50 percent and lost 25 percent of their weight, the men exhibited many similar behaviors.

As they lost weight, their food interest intensified. The men talked food, fantasized about food, collected recipes, studied cookbooks and menus, and developed odd eating rituals. They would dawdle up to two hours over a meal, toying with their food, cutting it in small pieces, adding spices, sometimes in distasteful ways, trying to make it seem like more and of more variety. They were possessive about food, hoarded food, and spent much time planning, preparing and eating food saved from meals. They ate their allotted food to the last crumb and licked their plates. They became angry when they saw others wasting food.

Feelings related to this kind of behavior are explained by a woman who had recovered from anorexia nervosa and bulimia nervosa, in *Eating Disorders.*

"While anorexic, my body not only anticipated eating, it reveled in it. Being starved and hungry makes the experience of eating more intense — almost sensual. The feeling is analogous to what is experienced when drinking water when extremely thirsty, sleeping after being totally exhausted, or urinating after one's bladder has become overly full. What is usually somewhat ordinary becomes exciting — something to look forward to in an otherwise painful and lonely world. This made changing behaviors so that I no longer experienced intense hunger extremely difficult."[17]

Risks of eating disorders

- Severe emotional and psychological changes
- Anemia
- Stomach cramping
- Electrolyte imbalance
- Tooth decay
- Bone fractures
- Stunted growth
- Cardiac arrhythmias
- Amenorrhea
- Kidney damage
- Death

Yet restoring full nutrition brings dramatic improvement to both the mind and body for sufferers of anorexia nervosa, as it did for Keys' volunteers.

Other eating disorders

Some eating disorders don't fit clearly into diagnostic criteria. They may have many of the features of anorexia or bulimia, but involve different eating behaviors, such as repeatedly chewing and spitting out, but not swallowing, large amounts of food.

Binge eating disorder is included in this group. This newly-identified disorder meets the criteria for bulimia nervosa except that individuals do not regularly engage in purging behavior and do not meet the criteria for being unduly concerned with weight and shape.

They eat large amounts of food, at least twice a week, in a relatively short time, with a sense of loss of control. They may be average weight, but most often are overweight.

This disorder was first described in 1959, and is similar to what has been called "compulsive eating." Research on binge eating is still in its infancy.

Excessive exercise

One of the fastest growing eating disorder behaviors in the past five years is excessive exercise or exercise addiction to lose weight or sculpt the body, says McVoy. Many anorectic and bulimic patients deal with some form of exercise dependency, explains Karin Kratina, MA, RD, an exercise physiologist and registered dietitian at the Renfrew Center in Florida.[18]

Excessive exercise aimed at weight loss is regarded as a secondary dependency, usually to an eating disorder, says Kratina. Physical activity takes priority over everything else for the exercise-dependent individual. He or she follows stereotyped patterns, continues exercising even when it causes or aggravates a serious physical disorder. When the person stops exercising, he or she experiences severe withdrawal symptoms.

"Stress injuries are common, and frequently the person exercises right through an injury so it can't heal properly," says Kratina.

Body sculpting entails exercise with the sole aim of spending calories to get rid of body fat in order to change body appearance. Body sculpting is intended to reduce body fat to a minimum, so the muscles can be more clearly defined, says McVoy.

"This has become more epidemic because of the growth in our society of an emphasis on fitness and body shaping. There's a great increase in fitness and muscle magazines, fitness spas, and home exercise equipment all with a focus on shape and muscle building."

Muscle and bodybuilding magazines for both men and women promote long hours of high-intensity exercise, and diets that are almost fat-free. The goal in competitive bodybuilding, written about endlessly, is to get "ripped," depleting almost all fat from between skin and muscle, and dehydrating so severely the skin is thin as paper. This defines the muscles, rope-like, and makes blood vessels stand out like veined leaves just under the skin's surface.

With these extreme efforts to reshape the body, it can be expected there is great potential for abuse. The emphasis in these magazines is on appearance, not improved skill or strength. Eating disorder specialists suggest that many women are substituting body-building for eating disorders, or combining the two.

Anorexia and bodybuilding have many similarities, points out David Schlundt, PhD, an eating disorder specialist at Vanderbilt University in Nashville. "There are special diets, use of diuretics, steroid use, obsessive exercise, very low fat diets, and so on. An obsession with changing size and shape of the body leads to extreme and sometimes dangerous changes in diet, exercise and substance abuse."[19]

One of the reasons eating disorders are increasing among young men is apparently a result of this obsession with muscles and body sculpting, reflecting their dissatisfaction with their natural bodies and an intense desire to change it, McVoy says.

Links to sexual abuse, violence

Childhood abuse of all kinds — sexual, physical, psychological, both subtle and dramatic — violates the boundaries of the self. These are invasions that can have extremely harmful effects. Violence, trauma and childhood sexual abuse are considered to be risk factors for developing eating disorders.

Sexual abuse is a common experience for many eating disorder patients, says Susan Wooley, PhD, a professor of psychology and co-director of the Eating Disorders Clinic at the University of Cincinnati Medical College.[20]

Until very recently, the importance of a history of sexual or physical abuse was minimized by the mostly-male therapists who dominated the field in research publishing and conference agendas. Wooley calls it the "concealed debate" which took place in conference hallways and is finally being recognized.

The National Women's Study, a national random sample of 4,008 adult women in the U.S. who were interviewed at least three times over the course of one year, found that women with bulimia nervosa were twice as likely to have been raped (27 percent vs 13 percent) or sexually molested (22 vs 12 percent), and four times likely to have experienced aggravated assault (27 vs 8 percent), compared to women without an eating disorder.

Overall, the majority of those with bulimia reported a lifetime history of some type of criminal victimization event compared to less than one-third of women who did not have an eating disorder (54 to 31 percent).

Twelve percent of women with bulimia nervosa had been raped as children, age 11 or younger, compared with 5 percent of women without an eating disorder. The age at the time of rape predated the age of the first binge episode in all cases, suggesting that childhood sexual abuse is a risk factor for bulimia, said the researchers.[21]

Even so, the true extent of sexual abuse is unknown due to the silencing of the victims, and their reluctance to disclose abuse even to therapists trained to help them in this area. Wooley cites one report that 33 percent of patients who later disclosed their abuse, had denied it during five weeks of hospitalization at a center highly experienced in abuse treatment and sensitized to its importance.

Another of the few clear findings of the past decade is the extremely long delay that may precede disclosure even among patients in extensive therapy, says Wooley.

She says underestimation is virtually unavoidable, yet critics express most concern with overestimation, despite lack of evidence for the latter and abundant evidence for the former. The accusation that the patient or therapist made it up holds sexual abuse to a test not customarily applied to clinical data, she charges.

Wooley reports the predominantly female patients more often disclose histories of sexual abuse to female than to male therapists. Most male therapists did not realize the extent and consequences of the abuse until recently. Now that it is recognized, she says there is a polarization over how to deal with it in the eating disorder field. The controversy involves whether to rely on medical or sociocultural models, on technical or humanistic approaches, apolitical or feminist analyses.

Wooley notes that the unmasking of sexual abuse was largely due to the efforts of feminist writers and clinicians.

Freud's deliberate suppression of the discovery of sexual abuse was only revealed in the early 1980s. Before the 1970s the social institutions that now help female victims of sexual abuse and domestic violence did not exist. Childhood sexual abuse was believed to be rare and likely harmless.

Eating disorder specialists Mark Schwartz and Leigh Cohn say sexual abuse was estimated to be 1 in 1,000 in the 1960s by a major psychiatric textbook. By the 1980s many publications were reporting an incidence of 1 in 3 females and 1 in 7 males.

They suggest that male clinicians have sometimes needed not to

---

Eating Disorder Warning Signs

National Eating Disorders Organizations

Anorexia nervosa

- Significant or extreme weight loss (at least 15%, with no known medical illness)
- Reduces food intake
- Develops ritualistic eating habits such as:
     a: Cutting up meat into extremely small bites
     b. Chewing every bite a large number of times
- Denies hunger
- Becomes more critical and less tolerant of others
- Exercises excessively (hyperactive)
- When eating, chooses low to no fat and low calorie foods
- Says he/she is too fat, even when this is not true
- Has highly self-controlled behavior
- Does not reveal feelings

Bulimia Nervosa

- Makes excuses to go to the restoom after meals

(continued on page 78)

Binge eating disorder *(continued from page 77)*

- Has mood swings
- May buy large amounts of food and then suddenly it disappears
- Unusual swelling around the jaw
- Weight may be within normal range
- Frequently eats large amounts of food, often high in calories, (a binge) and does not seem to gain weight
- May decide to purchase large quantities of food and eat it on the spur of the moment
- Laxative or diuretic wrappers found frequently in the trash can
- Unexplained disappearance of food in the home or residence hall setting

Binge Eating Disorder

- Frequently eats a large amount of food that is larger than most people would eat during a similar amount of time
- Eats rapidly
- Eats to point that is uncomfortably full
- Often eats alone
- Shows irritation and disgust with self after overeating
- Does not use methods to purge

Additional signs of related eating disorders

- Makes excuses to skip meals and does not eat with others
- Develops a tendency to be perfect in almost everything
- Conversation is mostly focused on foods or around body shape
- Often hears other people's problems but does not share her own
- Is highly self-critical
- Worries about what others think
- Thinks about weight and body shape most of the day
- Begins to isolate more from friends and family
- The odor of vomit is in the bathroom regularly
- Repeatedly chews and spits out food — does not swallow large amounts of food
- May purge and yet not binge eat[2]

NOTE: The more warning signs a person has, the higher the probability that the person has or is developing an eating disorder.

NEDO 1994/AFRAID TO EAT 1997

know and not to see, in order to maintain their own illusions. "The fundamental question is: Why has it taken so long to recognize the association if, as has been reported by one major center, 80 percent of their sample of eating-disordered patients have a history of sexual abuse? Why then has there been such resistance to knowing and believing?"

This information is all so new that there is wide variation in reports. It needs further investigation to clarify definitions, what should be considered sexual abuse, how to cope with the difficulty of disclosure, and how it can be assessed in a reliable way.

At the same time it needs to be recognized that some eating-disordered clients were not sexually or physically abused, and many sexually abused youngsters do not develop eating disorders.

If you're a girl, you have to be thin

While eating disorders are defined specifically in psychiatric texts, there appears to be a continuum of disordered eating, especially among women, write Patricia Fallon, Melanie Katzman and Wooley, editors of *Feminist Perspectives on Eating Disorders.*[22]

Some children, particularly girls, may be more vulnerable to dieting than others. Factors that increase a dieter's vulnerability to eating disorders are believed to be genetic, biological, psychological, sociocultural and familial, as well as having a history of sexual or physical abuse.

The traditional, patriarchal view suggests the roots for eating disorders lie with psychological traits of patients and their families.

But society has to take responsibility for the tremendous impact of persistent and pervasive cultural images of the desirable body.

In less than two decades, the acceptable female body size has been whittled down by one-third, say Fallon, Wooley and Katzman. Most women no longer fit that size, and trying to do so takes up more and more of their lives. Some are pushed to an apparent point of no return, say these eating disorder authorities, by "our era's culminating demand that women give up nourishment and a large share of their bodies."

For girls entering adolescence, accepting their rapidly-changing bodies becomes nearly impossible when placed against this cultural backdrop. Not only are their female role models extremely thin and usually dieting, but males they know are often openly admiring thin women and denigrating large women.

However, much progress has been made in the last decade in male therapists recognizing the conflicting messages adolescent girls are given in modern culture today.

Steven Levenkron, MS, author of *The Best Little Girl in the World,* suggests male therapists can be more effective if they are "parental" rather than "paternalistic" in their feelings toward patients.

"I don't think that there is anything problematic about men treating women with eating disorders if they understand the dilemma many women face in today's culture. This dilemma concerns how much to value their femininity while maintaining a level of assertiveness in order to compete with men."[23]

Others say they have learned how important it is to be silent and listen to girls and women, without taking the role of "male expert."

"Many if not most of the patients we treat have been traumatized either physically, sexually or simply in relationships where they've experienced some disappointment in others," says Craig L. Johnson, a clinical psychologist and co-director of the eating disorders program at the Laureate Psychiatric Clinic in Tulsa.[24]

See Appendix for Mental and Physical Complications of Eating Disorders.

CHAPTER 5

Size prejudice
punishes large children

■

Large children and teens often live with vicious prejudice from their classmates, parents and teachers — attitudes which can interfere with their ability to grow into self-assured, successful adults.

Research confirms what we all know, that there is strong prejudice against obese youngsters regardless of age, sex, race and socio-economic status. Many struggle with discrimination in education, employment, health care and social relationships.

Even young children feel the stigma of obesity and fear being a target. In one study children as young as 6 described silhouettes of an overweight child as "lazy, dirty, stupid, ugly, cheats and lies."

When shown drawings of a normal weight child, an overweight child, and children with various handicaps, including missing hands and facial disfigurement, children rated the overweight child as the least likable. Sadly, this bias even afflicted the larger children themselves, and they felt the same prejudices.[1]

Large children and teens can be healthy, eat normally and live active lives. But the stigma may be overwhelming, and it may be difficult for them to develop confident, healthy attitudes about themselves because of the devastating prejudice practiced by their peers, their parents and their teachers.

"Clearly obese children are blamed for their condition. It is an unusual person who does not fashion this into serious self-doubt and a persistent concern with dieting," says Kelly D. Brownell, an obesity researcher and professor of psychology at Yale University.[2]

Prejudice against large children may evolve into a form of persecution. They are teased on the playground, called names and are among the last chosen to play on teams.

But it is at puberty when the problems of obesity become most painful. Despite the discrimination against them, studies show that their sense of self-worth is similar for large children and average weight children. But by adolescence, the social messages become internalized and a lifelong negative self-image may develop, according to William Dietz and Nevin Scrimshaw, in Social Aspects of Obesity.[3]

Gaining a strong sense of self-worth is especially difficult for large teenagers in industrially developed countries, where in recent decades both feminine and masculine ideals have become very thin, and stars of movies, television, sports and pop music are not only lean, but males look well muscled and physically fit.

"All this results in a distressing position for an obese adolescent who has to face up to the negative attitudes of colleagues at school or even in the family. Clumsiness, unattractiveness to the opposite sex, are serious problems at this age," they note.

Obesity is the last socially acceptable form of prejudice, charge Albert Stunkard and Jeffery Sobal, writing in the text Eating Disorders and Obesity: "Obese persons remain perhaps the only group toward whom social derogation can be directed with impunity."[4]

Teachers can stop or reinforce prejudice

Discrimination has been shown in the way teachers interact with large students and the grades they give for comparable work. Acceptance into prestigious colleges is lower in one study for large females, even when they do not differ in academic qualifications, school performance or applications rates to colleges.[5]

But support for large children has come, somewhat unexpectedly, from the nation's largest teacher organization — the professionals who see size prejudice daily and potentially have the most power to bring about changes in how large children are treated.

The National Education Association (NEA) undertook a yearlong investigation into size discrimination against students and teachers in the schools as a human rights and civil rights issue.

In 1994 NEA published its 27-page "Report on Size Discrimination," which describes size discrimination in schools at every level and recommends follow-up action.[6]

The report says the school experience is one of "ongoing prejudice, unnoticed discrimination and almost constant harassment" for large students, and "socially acceptable yet outrageous insensitivity and rudeness" for large teachers.

"At the elementary level, children learn that it is acceptable to dislike and deride fatness. From nursery school through college, fat students experience ostracism, discouragement, and sometimes violence. Often ridiculed by their peers and discouraged by even well-meaning education employees, fat students develop low self-esteem and have limited horizons. They are deprived of places on honor rolls, sports teams, and cheerleading squads and are denied letters of recommendation."

A member of the school investigating team sympathized with large teens who are uncomfortable in showers and don't want other students to stare at or ridicule them. Another told of a high school drill team that for 10 years excluded overweight girls from the team. Those who were progressing toward their goal weight were allowed to practice at school but not perform in public.

My friend Carol Johnson, a Wisconsin therapist who founded Largely Positive support groups for large women, writes in her book, *Self-Esteem Comes in All Sizes,* how her cheerleading ambitions came to an abrupt end.

"One of my dreams was to be a cheerleader. When tryouts were announced in the seventh grade, I signed up immediately and practiced night and day. After tryouts, I knew I had given a flawless performance. However, the physical education teacher who was judging the competition took me aside and gently told me that although I was one of the best candidates, she simply could not choose me.

The reason? I was too chubby. My body was unacceptable for public display.

"Shortly thereafter, I became intrigued by the baton and decided to take twirling lessons. You would have thought the cheerleader episode would have deterred me forever, but somehow it didn't. I dreamed of leading the marching band down the football field, and adept as I was, I thought there was good chance this dream would become reality. Reality did set in, but not the one I had dreamed about. Once again I was trying to do something chubby girls weren't supposed to do — put themselves on display. This time I was told not to bother because the uniforms wouldn't fit me. I didn't even try out. And the message pierced deeper: You're not acceptable.

"The truth is that my weight in high school exceeded the weight charts by no more than 30 pounds. Now, when I look at my high school pictures, I don't think I look at all heavy. Yet at the time those extra 30 pounds felt like the weight of the world on my shoulders. Losing weight had become the most important thing in my life.

Carol says her parents always were always loving, supportive and proud of her, but they couldn't protect her from the outside world. "I truly believed, deep in my heart that I was not as good as the thinner girls. Only by losing weight could I become their equal."[7]

The NEA report quotes a New York Times article as an example of "outrageous behavior" to which large children are subjected in schools.

Aleta Walker never had any friends during her childhood and adolescence in Hannibal, Mo. Instead she was ridiculed and bullied every day. When she walked down the halls at school, boys would flatten themselves against the lockers and cry, "Wide load!"

But the worst was lunchtime, she said. "Every day there was this production of watching me eat lunch." She tried to avoid going to the school cafeteria. "I would hide out in the bathroom. I would hide out behind the gym by the baseball diamond. I would hide in the library."

One day, schoolmates started throwing food at her as she sat at a table at lunch. Plates of spaghetti splashed onto her face, and the long greasy strands dripped onto her clothes.

"Everyone was laughing and pointing. They were making pig

noises. I just sat there," she said.

Another friend of mine through the size acceptance movement is Cheri Erdman, now a 42-year-old therapist and college teacher. She was actually sent away from home at age 5, on the advice of a kindergarten teacher, to live for more than a year in a residential weight treatment facility for children with "special nutritional needs." In her book, *Nothing to Lose: A Guide to Sane Living in a Larger Body,* Erdman, describes the sadness of being separated from her family for so long.[8]

No safe haven at home

For some children, teasing and ridicule comes from inside the family circle, so there is no escape from tormentors. Pat, 34, describes her father's disdain of her size in *Real Women Don't Diet.*

"My experience of prejudice for being fat started at a very young age. The sadness and teasing I went through then was not from individuals outside my family; it was from within my family, by the people who are supposed to most love you. At the age of nine, I did not consider myself overweight, but in my father's opinion I was not only overweight but also a 'fat cow' and a 'fat pig.' His ridicule and teasing continued to tolerate the hatefulness of my classmates calling me 'fat Pat,' but then I would go home and hear my father threaten to send me to Missouri. He wanted to have his mom lock me up and feed me bread and water so that I could lose weight.

"My father's threats were always at the tip of his tongue. One time he had a new idea: 'If I tie you to the back of my truck and make you run around the block a few times, you'll really lose weight.' although he never did it, just the horror of knowing it might happen was never far away. During all the years of growing up, I never was able to defend myself. I felt like I was a leper or something very bad, just for being overweight. I spent years taking drugs. I overdosed many times. Why should I care? My life wasn't worth that much. After all, I was different. I was fat.[9]

Effects of this stigma carry over into adulthood, especially for women, reports Dietz.

Women who are overweight as adolescents or young adults

earn less, are less likely to marry, complete fewer years of school, and have higher rates of poverty than their normal weight peers. Few of these effects occur among overweight males.[10]

One study shows adults who were overweight as children, but of normal weight as adolescents, had a body image comparable to that of individuals who had never been overweight. But adults who had been obese as adolescents had an extremely negative body image and feelings of low self-worth.

Some of them experience a great deal of unresolved anger and rage. Jean Rubel, 36, describes turning this anger against herself.

"Under my loneliness simmered a lake of molten rage. Sometimes I turned it loose when I felt ignored, criticized, misunderstood, or unloved. Most of the time, though, I held it in the pit of my stomach, where it became the only defense I could find against my belief that I was flawed in some critical way that kept me from joining the human race. Unfortunately, I too often turned this hateful energy against myself in storms of self-criticism and loathing. I began to blame my body for all my problems. If I weren't so ugly, so big, so soft and flabby, I would be happy and popular. I was six feet tall and 145 pounds. According to yearbook pictures I was slender and reasonably attractive, but I couldn't see it. I wanted to be thin, admired, and loved. Instead I felt awkward, shy, fat, defective and extremely lonely."[11]

Charisse Goodman recounts the unfairness of her childhood experiences in *The Invisible Woman*.

"I was always 'the fat kid.' I wasn't me. I wasn't a name or a person, just an object described by an adjective. If I was naturally shy, I became doubly so.

"To make things worse, my family moved several times during my childhood. I found out early that I'd be lucky to have one or two friends who didn't care what I looked like. I learned that no matter what anyone says, it really doesn't county if you're smart, kind, funny, sweet, generous, or caring because you also happen to be heavy, you may find yourself on the receiving end of more cruelty than you even knew existed.

"I learned that keeping to myself and minding my own business didn't help because people would seek me out to ridicule and humiliate me. I learned that "ignoring it," as I was nonchalantly advised to do by my emotionally disengaged parents, usually just made me a great challenge to bullies, so that I inevitably became "the one to get." I learned that adults are often indifferent to the suffering of a fat child, perhaps because on some level they agree with her tormentors, or maybe it's just convenient for them to believe that an abused child will somehow emerge unscathed into adulthood, magically free of emotional scars.

"I discovered that anytime I moved my body, people would laugh at me, and that even if I sat still and quietly read a book they would point and laugh. I learned that if they saw me cry or show any weakness, they would laugh at me even more. And so I learned to cry alone, and laugh alone, and live alone inside my head. I learned that the word "pretty" never included me.

"Even those times when I lost weight to try and fit in, it was never enough, and I grew to realize that when it was time to choose teammates for a game, or dates for a dance, I was invisible; but when someone needed a cheap laugh or a quick ego boost at my expense, people saw me, all right. I learned my place. I tried to learn not to care.

"As I grew up, I assumed a stone-faced mask in order to deprive people of their sickening delight in hurting me, a mask which in later years I would find extremely difficult to remove. I became a tense child with a perpetual air of bewilderment. But I was not angry. Any anger on my part was met by adults with the huffy insistence that I had a hostility problem. What other people did to me was natural and normal, while I was neither.

"Now I am a grown woman. I know without a doubt that in every town and every city, in every state in America, countless other fat children are learning the same heartbreaking, soul-destroying lessons that I was forced to learn. My pain and the pain of others like me has been conveniently invisible to thin people for far too long. They have been too comfortable with the price that we have paid for their imaginary superiority.

"At long last, I am angry."[12]

Venting feelings

Nancy Summer, another friend and leader in the size acceptance movement, brings workshops in antiviolence, anti-prejudice programs to sixth-grade girls.

She encourages the girls to vent their worst prejudices against large people and get all the negative things out in the open right away.

"I invite them to insult me. 'What do you think when you see a person as fat as me? What words come to mind? You can be honest.' (I weigh more than 400 pounds.)

"After the initial giggling and squirming in chairs, the responses are never the same. In one class, a rambunctious thin girl looks me dead in the eye and calls me a horse! 'Good!' I say. I smile and write horse on the flip chart and then ask if they can think of other animals that are associated with fat people. Soon horse is joined by suggestions from other girls: cow, elephant, pig, hippo, buffalo, and whale. Then we discuss how beautiful these animals are in their own right. My calm response to the challenge sets the tone for that workshop.

"Whether the girls are polite or candid, aware of the issues or not, we always manage to bring out many of the stereotypes and negative language that they've heard (and use) about fat people. They especially enjoy talking about their larger teachers in a setting where they can 'get away with it.' One girl actually admits that she teased a teacher until she made her cry. She is proud of this revelation until she hears her classmates define this as being mean.

"When a group is too polite, I ask what the boys say to or about fat girls, and that often brings lots of responses: 'Shamu,' 'bubble butt,' and 'lard ass' are favorites. We also discuss the many stereotypes people believe about fat kids and adults. 'Fat and lazy,' 'Fat people eat all the time,' and 'Boys don't think fat girls are pretty' are just some of the responses I get. I always counter the negative stereotypes with facts and personal stories. For example, when one girl says that fat people are stupid, I counter with the fact that when I was in sixth grade, I was invited into a program where I could skip eighth grade.

"But always I stress my basic message: bias against fat hurts people of all sizes. 'Imagine that you are sitting in the lunchroom and a bully starts making fun of a fat kid a few tables away. How does that make you feel?' I ask them. 'We can imagine that the fat kid feels bad about being picked on, but what about all the other kids who hear it?'

"I'd be afraid he'd pick on me next," one girl responds. Another says, "I'd be afraid that if I got fat, people would pick on me, too." " I wouldn't eat my dessert." "I'd probably laugh, too," one candid soul admits, but goes on to tell us about a fat boy in her school who always laughs when people pick on him. One brave girl says, "I'd tell him to shut up."

"I explain that it isn't just large kids and adults who are hurt by size discrimination. Everyone else is hurt, too, because as long as fat is hated, everyone will be afraid of becoming fat. Fear of fat makes everyone unhappy and dissatisfied with their bodies. And that makes us have lower self-esteem and less self-confidence. And sometimes it can lead to dangerous diets and eating disorders."

Clearly size prejudice is a potent force for these youngsters and 6th grade girls understand it well.

Educators and health professionals need to be aware of the size prejudice encountered by these young people as they work with them to develop normal eating and healthy living.

"At the elementary level, children learn that it is accept-able to dislike and deride fatness. From nursery school through college, fat students experience ostracism, discouragement, and sometimes violence. Often ridiculed by their peers and discouraged by even well-meaning education employees, fat students develop low self-esteem and have limited horizons. They are deprived of places on honor rolls, sports teams, and cheerleading squads and are denied letters of recommendation."

THE NATIONAL EDUCATION ASSOCIATION
REPORT ON SIZE DISCRIMINATION IN SCHOOLS, 1994

CHAPTER 6

Overweight rates
keep rising

■

What is obesity? When is a child overweight and what causes it?

These are old questions and yet ones so new that before 1980, many believed obesity to be simply a problem of too many calories. As a result, the solutions offered by experts were equally simplistic — and claimed to be effective even when they weren't.

Now, scientists around the world are studying these urgent questions and many others: What are the hallmarks of obesity? Does it start in childhood, through excess fat cell development, or even in the womb? Is it most likely to be triggered at high-risk points during a child's development? How powerful are genetic factors? And if they are important determinants of obesity, why are we seeing such steep increases in just the past decade?

While there have been advances, much remains unknown and the subject of intense debate. The bottom line is that researchers and many health professionals now recognize obesity as a prevalent and complex condition that resists intervention. The fact is, there is much we don't know about childhood obesity — most importantly what to do about it.

"Obesity continues to humble the scientific community by eluding effective understanding and intervention in many important respects," says Shiriki Kumanyika, associate professor of nutrition epidemiology at Pennsylvania State University.

Prevalence

While researchers and health professionals ponder childhood overweight and its causes and outcomes, one thing is clear: The prevalence has increased sharply for both children and adolescents in the U.S. in the last decade as found in the latest NHANES III study *(fig. 1)*. Not only are more youngsters overweight, but they are more severely overweight than ever before.

Some recent landmark studies reveal the striking evidence. NHANES III, one of the largest health studies showed that 22 percent of kids ages 6 to 17 are overweight — 7 percentage points more than in 1963. Additionally, the percent of children who are seriously overweight has more than doubled, growing from 5 percent to 11 percent for both girls and boys.

This study looked at 2,290 youth ages 6 to 17 and compared their body mass with children who were measured in 1963. It's one of the most comprehensive examinations of American youth, done by re-

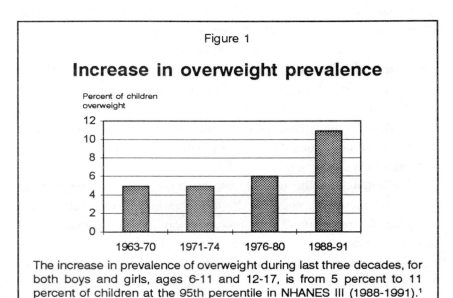

Figure 1

Increase in overweight prevalence

Percent of children overweight

The increase in prevalence of overweight during last three decades, for both boys and girls, ages 6-11 and 12-17, is from 5 percent to 11 percent of children at the 95th percentile in NHANES III (1988-1991).[1]

ARCH PEDIATR ADOLESC MED 1995/AFRAID TO EAT 1997

searchers at the National Center for Health Statistics at the Centers for Disease Control and Prevention in Hyattsville, Md.

An overweight child fell into the 85th percentile, defined as a body mass index of 23 at ages 12-14; 24 at ages 15-17 and 26 at ages 18-19. To arrive at this definition, cutoff points were set in 1963-65 at the top weight of 85 percent of children in each age group. Thus, by definition, 15 percent of children were overweight at that time; 22 percent now *(fig. 2)*.

A seriously overweight child fell into the 95th percentile, a controversial category and the recommended cutoff point for younger children ages 6 to 11. By narrowing the definition of overweight or seriously overweight to the 95th percentile, growing children can have a wider range of weight and fat changes without being categorized or stigmatized as overweight.

What alarms public health officials is that rates of overweight were fairly stable for children and teens during the 1960s and 1970s, but during the 1980s, both children and adults gained weight. The same study found that the number of overweight adults had changed from one in four to one in three during the same decade.[1]

In the face of these trends, the goal of Healthy People 2000 to

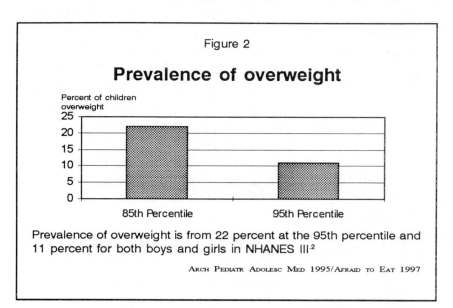

Figure 2

Prevalence of overweight

Percent of children overweight

85th Percentile   95th Percentile

Prevalence of overweight is from 22 percent at the 95th percentile and 11 percent for both boys and girls in NHANES III.[2]

Arch Pediatr Adolesc Med 1995/Afraid to Eat 1997

reverse the prevalence of overweight to 15 percent or less for children and adolescents by the century's end is impossible.

Another study that documents the same growth in overweight among children is the Bogalusa Heart Study. During the past 14 years, this survey of 2,500 to 3,500 youth has measured dramatic increases in overweight among children ages 5 to 14.[2] At each age level, children were heavier by 5.5 pounds in 1984 than they were in 1973. However, whether or not children gained weight seemed to be related to their baseline weight. Lean kids tended to remain lean, and those who were overweight initially had gained the most weight. But the researchers couldn't find that the heavier children were eating more. They surmise that the heavier kids may be less active.

Higher rates for minorities

More minority children seem to be overweight than their white peers, the NHANES III study shows (fig. 3). In the narrowest category of

Figure 3

Prevalence of overweight

NHANES III

Sex, Age and Race-Ethnicity[3]

	Percentile	
Category	85th	95th
Boys aged 6-11		
Total	21.9	11.3
Non-Hispanic white	20.5	10.4
Non-Hispanic black	26.5	13.4
Mexican American	33.3	17.7
Boys aged 12-17		
Total	22.0	12.8
Non-Hispanic white	23.1	14.4
Non-Hispanic black	21.1	9.3
Mexican American	26.7	12.8
Girls aged 6-11		
Total	22.7	10.6
Non-Hispanic white	21.5	9.8
Non-Hispanic black	31.4	16.9
Mexican American	29.0	14.3
Girls aged 12-17		
Total	21.4	8.8
Non-Hispanic white	20.3	8.3
Non-Hispanic black	29.9	14.4
Mexican American	23.4	8.7

ARCH PEDIATR ADOLESC MED VOL 149, OCT 1995/
AFRAID TO EAT 1997

overweight, the 95th percentile, here's how children ages 6 to 11 ranked:

- African American: boys - 13 percent; girls - 17 percent
- Mexican-American: boys - 18 percent; girls - 14 percent
- White: boys, - 10 percent; girls - 10 percent

Rates for ages 12 to 17 at the 85th percentile reflect the same differences:

- African American: boys - 21 percent; girls - 30 percent
- Mexican-American: boys - 27 percent; girls - 23 percent
- White: boys, - 23 percent; girls - 20 percent

Black children, especially, are not only heavier, but taller and mature earlier. Even at age 10, black girls were 11 pounds heavier, 1.6 inches taller and had more body fat. And they reach puberty earlier, as a study of black Harlem youth shows. Children who are heavier often reach puberty early, apparently as a result of higher body fat.[3]

Overweight is especially high among some American Indian children. Rates range from 40 percent to 50 percent, depending on the study and the tribe.[4] A look at Zuni children found that more than half of girls and a third of boys ages 11 to 20 were overweight. Interestingly, a study of Cherokee teens found that trend reversed — half of boys and one in four girls.[5]

The Pima people, which have struggled with extremely high rates of diabetes, also seem to have children who are taller, heavier and have more body fat than white children of the same age. One study of Pima youth shows about half exceed the 95th percentile of weight-for-age. Again, their increased height may be explained by faster growth and early puberty.[6]

Fat patterning and body composition

How fat is distributed on the body can indicate what health problems children are at risk for. If the fat is concentrated around the abdomen, they may have a greater chance of developing cardiovascular disease and other problems at a younger age.[7]

Ethnicity or race may determine a child's build and fat patterning. Black and Mexican American children tend to have more ab-

Figure 4

Overweight definition

as used in NHANES III

Age (years)	BOYS		GIRLS	
	Height (inches)	Weight (pounds)	Height (inches)	Weight (pounds)
6	47	56	47	57
8	51	75	52	80
10	56	96	56	104
12	60	123	61	137
14	66	164	63	151
16	69	183	65	173

Average heights by year of age and weight that correspond to the definition of overweight at the 95th percentile, as defined from NHES II and III. Overweight is defined as equal or greater than this level.[4]

TROIANO R P./AFRAID TO EAT 1997

dominal distribution of fat than white children, and this increases with age, particularly for boys, according to William Mueller of the School of Public Health, University of Texas Health Science Center who analyzed data on national and other studies of children and adolescents.[8]

Defining obesity

Currently, there is not a clearly accepted definition of overweight for children and adolescents, despite considerable use of the NHANES III 85th and 95th percentile cutoff points. This definition provides the cutoff points shown (*fig. 4*). Another definition being used is based on body fat, defining as obese a level of 25 percent or more for boys and 30 percent or more for girls.[9]

Other specialists say that more factors need to be considered, such as family history to determine what is a normal weight for a child. Whether because of genetics or family practices, the assessment of obesity must involve the family as well as the individual youngster, says the California position paper "Children and Weight:

A Changing Perspective," by Eileen B. Peck, DrPH, RD, and Helen D. Ullrich, MA, RD.

"Do we really need a definition of childhood obesity?" asks Katherine M. Flegal, PhD, Chief Medical Statistics Branch, Division of Health Examination Statistics at the National Center for Health Statistics at the Centers for Disease Control and Prevention in Hyattsville, Md.

Putting children into medically-defined categories connected to levels of overweight or obesity will stigmatize them, she said. That's why Flegal and the other federal researchers reporting NHANES III findings are reluctant to label children. They're concerned that their statistics will be used aggressively in attempting to deal with obesity in children and adolescents. There are wide differences in the way children grow and develop at every age, and low calorie diets are not recommended for children.[10]

The terms overweight and obesity are often used interchangeably, as they are in this book, defined in a general way as any recognized degree of excess weight or body fat.

What happened?

Although we knew it was coming from the many smaller studies all pointing to increases in overweight, the NHANES III statistics sent a shock wave through the health community.

What happened? Why did obesity rates jump across the board for young and old, males and females, and for every ethnic and racial group during the last decade?

The nature of obesity is not well understood. The interplay of inherited tendencies, the thrifty gene of minorities, food supply, physical activity, culture, socioeconomic and psychological factors all have a profound effect on the regulation of appetite and how energy is used or stored as fat.

The tendency to gain excessive fatness varies from one person to another, even in the same family, and even when food intake, physical activity and lifestyle appear to be the same. Metabolism rate may play a part, but it's more complex than this. It is possible that for some individuals, genetic factors route more of the fat intake into

Ethnic differences in fat patterning

Ethnic differences in body build and fat patterning were analyzed by William Mueller of the School of Public Health, University of Texas Health Science Center, using data on national and other studies of children and adolescents.

His studies show ethnicity accounts for about one third to half of the variance of sex and maturation. Sex accounts for 10 to 15 percent of patterning differences, maturation about 17 percent, and ethnicity 5 percent, says Mueller.

His findings are independent of average fatness levels. However, Mueller suggests some of the variance may be the result of the differing obesity levels in black and Mexican American children.

Comparing statistics on black, Mexican American and white children, Mueller reports the following:

1. Children age 1 to 5
- Preschool children are much more peripheral in fat distribution (less centralized) than older children.
- Black preschool children have more centralized fat patterning than white preschoolers.

2. Adolescents
- Mexican American children have higher skinfold measures at triceps, subscparular and suprailiac, but lower at medial calf site, compared with white children; thus, theirs is an upper body obesity.
- Black children have lower skinfolds at both arm and leg sites than white children; their fat is more centrally distributed.

3. Girls age 12 to 17
- Fatness increases with age for all three groups.

- Black and Mexican American girls have a more central distribution of fat than white girls, who have more peripheral fat patterning.

4. Boys age 12 to 17
- Centrality of fat increases with age in all three groups.
- Black and Mexican American boys have a more centralized fat patterning than white boys.

5. Other differences, ages 6 to 17
- Black children tend to have more centralized fat patterning at all ages, with less arm and leg fat, compared with white children.
- Black children have the broadest shoulders and narrowest hips, compared with both Mexican and white children.
- Mexican American children have more upper body fatness with less leg fat, compared with white children.
- Mexican Americans tend to have the narrowest shoulders of the three groups.
- A sex difference emerges at puberty, but ethnic differences remain.
- Individuals with non-insulin dependent diabetes (ages 14 to 17) tend to have broader shoulders and narrower hips than nondiabetic individuals of same sex and age.
- Circumference ratios of waist-to-hip do not show the ethnic differences of skinfold data, although they show a consistent sex difference. Thus body circumferences in children may be measuring muscle and bone development, not fatness levels.[5]

Bouchard, Johnston, 1988.
Healthy Weight Journal, 1988.

storage, and that they have extraordinary ability, not only protect that stored fat, but to restore it quickly after it's been depleted from dieting or fasting.

Perhaps the simplest, most likely explanation is an increase in inactivity and sedentary living. Other potent factors: Women are having bigger babies today, encouraged by public health policies aimed at preventing low birth weights. But this may increase the legacy of overweight for both babies and teenage mothers. Also, there may be higher population increases in the socioeconomic groups and ethnic minorities with the "thrifty gene."

An easy answer to high weight gains is too much high-fat food, and certainly this is a factor for many youth today. Yet, on the average, children as well as adults are eating less fat today than a decade ago, and while there may be calorie increases, they appear to be small. Fat consumption has dropped from 36 to 34 percent of total calories in the last decade, although an increase in calories may mean there is no actual drop in total fat. However, current debate questions whether the decrease in fat and diet changes for children may be part of the problem. And obesity rates continue to increase.

Genetic factors

Family makes a difference. About 25 percent of adult obesity can be traced to genetic origin, with another 30 percent from family cultural factors, according to Claude Bouchard, PhD, a professor of exercise physiology at Laval University, Quebec, who has done extensive research with identical twins, reared apart and together, adoptees and their two sets of families, and nine types of relatives.[11]

Children, especially young children, are tremendously influenced by their families. A child of two overweight parents has an 80 percent chance of becoming overweight, compared with a 14 percent chance for the child of two normal weight parents.[12]

For children of African, American Indian, Mexican or Pacific Island descent, the "thrifty gene" theory helps explain why obesity rates are so high. The theory is that certain factors, such as storing fat efficiently, helped people survive under the harsh conditions of ancient times. People with these genes were most likely to survive and pass on efficient fat storage genes. But in a world abundant in high-fat food and sedentary living, having a thrifty gene that readily stores fat can be a disadvantage.[13]

Genetic factors may be associated with such regulators as basal metabolism, dietary thermogenesis, appetite, satiety, endocrine function and fat storage. Yet Bouchard cautions against putting too much emphasis on genetics. Many factors are involved, and there's "a lot of chaos in the body system we're working with," he says.

"We are probably overemphasizing the importance of genetics in obesity . . . We are seeing big increases in obesity worldwide — this has to be the result of environmental factors."

Inactivity

It's hard to measure physical activity, but most experts agree there's probably been a continuing decline.

Our streets are perceived as unsafe, so more children and youth stay indoors, watching television, playing video games and surfing the Internet. In today's climate of decreasing budgets, thousands of schools are cutting physical education programs. In 1995 only 25 percent of school children attended daily physical education class.

The more children watch television, the higher their risk for becoming overweight, no matter what their race. It may mean they are less active or snack more in front of the TV. Or television itself may have a direct effect in lowering metabolic rate, as one study found.

The time children spent watching television increased during the 1980s, as did the rates of overweight. In one study of the relationship between television and weight, which may also explain some racial differences, black girls watched 36 hours or more a week compared with 24 hours or more for white girls. Girls of both races who watched more television tended to be more overweight. Girls who said they usually ate while watching television had higher caloric intake than did those who did not. Almost twice as many black girls as white girls reported that they usually ate while watching television.[14]

Food intake

Less physical activity, more high-fat, high-calorie foods. Many researchers say this is the recipe for overweight children, even though large kids aren't necessarily eating more than their lean peers. It may be the kinds of food they're eating, higher-fat foods, especially foods such as crackers and chips — and less meat, eggs and milk.

A group of black and white girls ages 9 and 10 kept food diaries for three days and gave researchers an insight into the link between body composition, eating and exercise. The black girls, who tended to be heavier, ate more calories and fat than the white girls. They ate less meat, milk and cheese and snacked more on high-fat foods. They also watched more hours of television and videos per week, which seemed to be more directly related to overweight than the foods they ate. For white girls, eating high-fat foods and watching TV were directly related to overweight.

Also, more families are eating outside the home more often, and at restaurants where larger meals are being served than in the past.

Family control effects

What you do, what you say and how you eat in a family counts. Simple things, like urging a child to clear her plate can have a direct effect on overweight.

Fourteen families participated in a psychology study at North Dakota State University in Fargo. It found that overweight children between age 1 and 3 were urged to eat both verbally and nonverbally by their parent more than twice as often as normal weight children. Overweight children received an average of 43 prompts per meal compared with 18 for the normal weight children *(fig. 5)*. All the children usually ate more when prompted to do so. Parents prompted their children to eat with words or by giving them food one-fourth of the time. When a child refused food, almost nine out of 10 times the parents gave further prompts to eat, and 70 percent of the time, the child did then eat.

They concluded that many parents selectively encourage mealtime behaviors of their very young children in ways which lead directly to excess weight gain.[15]

On the other hand, children may also gain excess weight from being fed in a restrained fashion which does not satisfy their needs, reports Ellyn Satter.

Parents often believe that their children can't regulate their food intake and that it's their job as a parent to get their child to eat. But those strategies, intended to feed a child a well-balanced diet, can be coercive and controlling. Studies suggest that children as young as age 3 can regulate their own food intake and a controlling, authoritarian parenting style impedes children's ability to develop self-control.[16]

When parents focus too much on the meal, the time of day for meals or how much food is left on the plate, their children don't learn normal eating habits that respond to hunger and satiety. And a parent who is dieting may be too involved in the child's weight and eating habits and see that child at risk for obesity.

"We emphasize that it is important for parents to create an optimal environment for their children's growth and health by providing a variety of nutritious foods. It should remain within the child's domain, however, to maintain control over how much of these foods are eaten," advise the Illinois researchers.

Poor family communication may also contribute to overweight. If children are isolated in a disinterested or disengaged family, they may be at a higher risk of overweight, reports Laurel Mellin, MA, RD, San Francisco. Her study of 254 obese adolescents found that four factors accounted for most of the weight differences: family cohesion, adolescent communication, age of obesity onset and the mother's weight.

It was surprising, Mellin reports, that the major environmental factors were not diet and activity, but instead were related to relationships, family cohesion and communication. Thus obesity increased as families were less engaged and the adolescent less engaging. She suggests that targeting family interaction and teaching family interactional skills may have more effect on weight than targeting diet and physical activity alone.[17]

How obesity develops in infants

From birth, babies born to overweight mothers appear to be at a higher risk for becoming overweight. Studies of British and Canadian children show that even if the babies are normal weight at birth, by age 6 months they are growing faster and are heavier than other infants. However not all fat babies are at risk.[18]

Some researchers have observed that infants who are quiet, inactive and placid tend to become overweight even with moderate intakes of food.12 This may be considered normal.

A child's family, regular eating habits, exercise, but not necessarily food intake, seem to determine whether a baby will grow into an overweight child. A 16-year longitudinal study followed followed 180 children from age 6 months to age 16, in Berkeley, Calif. The type of infant feeding or when solid food was introduced made no difference. Neither did the kinds of food eaten for meals or snacks, or whether the child had a sweet tooth.[19]

Bigger babies

Since 1989, Public Health directives have called on women to produce larger babies (8 to 8.5 pounds) by gaining more weight in pregnancy, in a perplexing move to reduce the number of small, premature babies. Although this is a controversial issue, there is much recent evidence to suggest that the larger babies American women are having are more likely to be overweight later in life. This

Figure 5

Parental food prompts
per meal[6]

Average per child	Normal weight child	Overweight child
Encouragements to eat	4	16
Food presentations	11	20
Offers of food	3	7
Total food prompts	18	43

HEALTHY WEIGHT JOURNAL/ION REVIEWS 1988

may be especially true for minority children.

Ray Yip, MD, MPH, Centers for Disease Control, reports that data from the CDC surveillance programs show that birth weight influences subsequent growth. Heavy infants at birth are four times as likely to become heavy 5-year-olds, he told attendees at the Workshop on Child and Adolescent Obesity, University of Iowa, in 1993.[20]

Another federal analysis of effect of birth weight on height and weight showed similar results: children with higher birth weights were heavier and taller at age 6 to 11. Height may be related partly to earlier maturity.[21]

Infant feeding

Breastfeeding, when possible, seems to be a healthy course for both mothers and babies, but its association with weight is unclear. Some studies in the 1970s suggested that bottle-feeding and the early introduction of solid foods contributed to childhood obesity, but some more recent studies refute that claim.

A four-year study of babies in Maine found no relationship between formula feeding or the early introduction of solid foods and preschool obesity. Solid foods were given earlier to babies who were bottle-fed, while babies that were breastfed ate solid foods when they were older. Four years later, 12 percent of the children were considered overweight, but there was no relationship to feeding practices.[22]

Weight gain in pregnancy

Heavier girls with high levels of body fat enter puberty early, which not only increases their risk for overweight, but also increases their risk for pregnancy. In addition, these early teen and pre-teen mothers are urged to have heavier babies. Those who are poor and members of ethnic groups with high obesity rates face even more risk. Women have long recognized that weight gain in pregnancy is critical in triggering obesity, but it is still barely acknowledged by the medical and health communities. Many doctors shrug it off, saying the mother can always lose any excess weight later. Unfortunately, this is not true.

The problem of excessive weight gain in pregnancy is especially acute for minorities. There is evidence that African-American women normally gain less in pregnancy than white women and have smaller babies, who then grow faster in their early years than white babies. By age 1 to 4, growth is accelerated for black children over that of white children, according to Shiriki Kumanyika, PhD, professor of nutrition at Pennsylvania State University. Small babies are common in Africa, she says.[23]

American Indian babies, too, were known to be smaller in earlier times and childbirth was easier. It may be that this is a genetic survival trait. The insistence of public health policy that minority babies be large may not be as beneficial as expected, since it is paralleled by a steep increase in obesity for both minority women and their children.

At the same time, it is an urgent concern that many young pregnant girls are so poorly nourished, often from dieting, that they do not gain enough weight in pregnancy to support both a healthy growth of the infant and their own growth demands. Young girls have high rates of giving birth to very small, high-risk, premature babies.

Thus, it is important that pregnant teens and preteens receive early nutrition counseling and prenatal care.

Risks of overweight

* Children who are overweight may be at risk early for diabetes and cardiovascular problems that could track into adulthood. And since the social stigma of being large is so strong, they're also at risk for using dangerous weight loss methods or developing eating disorders. Increasingly, health problems resulting from unsafe weight loss and ill-advised treatment are being recognized as risks of being overweight for children as well as adults.

Overweight children tend to grow faster. They're taller earlier, their fat-free mass is larger, their bone ages are advanced, and puberty occurs earlier. At the same time, there are also serious concerns that overzealous interventions may interfere with children's normal growth and development.

The risks which are related specifically to adolescent obesity, as given by Pauline Powers, MD, at the NIH Strategy Development

Workshop for Public Education on Weight and Obesity, sponsored by the National Heart, Lung and Blood Institute, include these health risks:

- Increased blood pressure
- Increased total cholesterol and abnormal lipoprotein rations
- Hyperinsulinemia

She also includes these psychological risks:

- Poor body image, which is "imprinted" in adolescence
- Low self-esteem, including fear of obesity and increasing pre-occupation with size and shape
- Cultural stigmatization. Children and adults devalue overweight children.[24]

Being overweight as a child may influence adult health. Tufts University researchers found that men who were 20 pounds or more overweight as teenagers were twice as likely to have died or have heart disease by age 70. They were also more likely to suffer colon and rectal cancer and to develop gout. Risks were lower for those who were not overweight as adults than for the men who remained overweight throughout life. However, there was no added health risk at age 70 for women who were overweight as teens. They did have double the risk of arthritis, and eight times as much difficulty in walking a quarter of a mile, climbing stairs and lifting heavy objects. The study looked at health records of students and tracked their weights and health for 55 years. The researchers say the message is not to pressure overweight kids to diet, boys in particular, but to encourage all youngsters to make healthful eating and exercise habits a regular part of everyday life.[25]

The Bogalusa Heart Study a clustering of three risk factors was found to be highly correlated with obesity, especially with abdominal fat. The three risk factors were systolic blood pressure, fasting insulin, and ratio of low and very low density lipoprotein cholesterol to high density lipoprotein cholesterol. Children in the upper third of obesity had increased clustering, while lean children showed less clustering than expected. The Bogalusa team suggests the prevention of the onset of obesity in early life may be important in reducing coronary heart disease in later life.[26]

It should be noted that physical fitness is related to blood pressure in children, age 5 to 6, independent of obesity in both cross-sectional and longitudinal studies, reports Steven Shea, MD, Columbia Presbyterian Medical Center. Because of mobility or social reasons, some large children may tend to be sedentary.

Indeed, some childhood specialists suggest that the greatest health hazards to childhood obesity may be mental, emotional and social effects. They say the most serious effects may be psychological, being labelled and stigmatized as obese, and long-term damage to self-esteem, self-concept and body concept.[27] It is clear that obesity can be a severe social handicap for a child.

Others point out this is not a reason to change the child, but rather to change the culture.

Early puberty

Early puberty may be another, largely-unrecognized risk of obesity. This is a factor in the high rates of teenage pregnancy in the U.S. and may increase the risk of reproductive cancers later in life, says Rose Frisch, PhD, Harvard Center for Population Studies.[28]

The age of puberty for American and European boys and girls has been dropping steadily during the last 100 years, and there is evidence that high body fat and sedentary living are associated with this trend. Instead of reaching menarche at age 15 or 16 and their adult height at 20 to 21 years as they did 100 years ago, American girls now reach menarche at an average of 12.8 years and complete growth by age 16 to 18, according to Frisch's research. Mean weight at menarche is 105 pounds (47.8 kg) with about 22 percent body fat, says Frisch. Yet female athletes still average 15.5 years at menarche, about the same as a century ago.

"Children now are bigger sooner. And girls on the average reach the mean weight at menarche . . . more quickly," says Frisch.

Early puberty means girls can get pregnant sooner and it also may be related to higher rates of reproductive cancers later in life. Puberty onset is more closely related to size, weight and percent of body fat than to age, writes Frisch, in her 1990 book , *Adipose Tissue and Reproduction.*[29]

Average fat content is 25 to 30 percent for young adult females, according to the American Alliance for Health, Physical Education, Recreation and Dance, 1984.

Young women who exercise regularly, even train athletically, delay puberty by months, even years, Frisch says. In a study of female college athletes who began training before menarche, the average began having their periods at age 15, about three years later than women who began training after menarche.

Each year of premenarcheal athletic training delays menarche by five months, Frisch suggests, and this formula should be applied. "One constructive way to reduce the incidence of teenage pregnancy would be to have girls join teams at ages 8 to 9 years and maintain regular moderate exercise." She says this may also reduce the risk of serious diseases in later life.

Former college athletes have a lower lifetime risk of breast cancer and other cancers of the reproductive system. Frisch studied 5,398 former college athletes and non-athletes ages 20 to 80. The most likely explanation for the reduced risk among athletes, Frisch says, is that they had lower levels of estrogen because they were leaner, and more of the estrogen was metabolized to the nonpotent catechol estrogens. "These data indicate that longterm exercise which was not Olympic or marathon level, but moderate and regular, reduces the risk of sex hormone-sensitive cancers, and the risk of diabetes for women later in life."

At the same time, it is critical that female athletes eat well and are fully nourished to avoid risk to their bones.

Tracking obesity

One of the more controversial issues in determining what to do about childhood obesity is what impact it has on later life. Does obesity track into adulthood? Is the child charting a course that will lead to lifelong obesity and perhaps related health risks, which might have been altered by making early changes?

Or will young children outgrow their fatness? If they do, being wrongly identified as obese may contribute to psychosocial difficulties, and growth may be affected by weight loss attempts. Two important factors to consider are the severity and age of the youngster. Severe obesity at any age is probably likely to continue.

Yet it is important to recognize that most large infants and pre-school children will probably outgrow their fatness. Interfering may distort a child's natural growth and development. But obesity at age 10 or 12, and especially during adolescence, is more likely to persist into adulthood.

In a University of Iowa study, well over half of children and teens who were in the highest of five weight categories, remain in this same category as adults. But nearly one-third dropped to the lower three quintiles.[30]

The following data compiled by Leonard Epstein, PhD, from four epidemiological studies, shows the likelihood of obesity tracking into adulthood, based on age:

Age of obese child	Percent who become obese adults	Relative risk
0- 6 months	14	2.3
6 months - 5.5 years	20	3.4
7 years	41	3.7
10-12 years	70	6.0

The risk of the overweight child becoming an overweight adult increases with age.[31]

He says this suggests ages when interventions might be helpful.

Yet it also indicates the importance of not overreacting. It shows about 60 percent of youngsters who are obese even at age 7 will not be obese as adults.

Adolescence

Dietz says obesity that began in adolescence tends to be more severe than is adult-onset obesity, and that most adults with severe obesity were overweight as adolescents. This is especially true for women. About one-third of all adult obesity in women began in adolescence, he notes, and he believes obesity in women is less likely to change than it is for men.[32]

Some overweight teens are more likely to become overweight adults if they exhibit certain factors: genetic predisposition; less sodium pump activity which apparently makes more fat available for storage; defects in temperature regulation; more active lipoprotein lipase; hyperinsulinemia, which tends to maintain the obese state; less thermogenesis; adipocyte hypertrophy and hyperplasia; and sex differences in body fat distribution.

Psychological factors that may contribute to maintaining obesity longterm include body image disturbances, low self-esteem and stigmatization, she suggests, because they may make it more difficult to lose or stabilize weight.[33]

CHAPTER 7

Lifestyle choices
increase problems

■

The problem of unhealthy eating goes far beyond the dinner table. So do the problems of a sedentary lifestyle. How children learn to eat and the activity habits they develop now can affect them the rest of their lives.

In Canada, kids and adults are encouraged to "eat well, live actively and feel good about yourself," clearly the best way to prevent weight and eating problems.

But we in the United States don't get that message. And the results are very disturbing, shocking even. After several decades of teaching children and families about healthy living, I was appalled, but hardly surprised, by recent reports that many American girls are malnourished.

The startling truth is that most teenage girls do not eat enough for health, energy and strength. They are discouraged from competing in sports. And they feel so bad about themselves that one-third report having seriously considered suicide in the past 12 months — double the rates of boys their age.

What is the problem? Why are so many girls disheartened? Why are so many malnourished and undernourished, starving in the midst of plenty?

What foods?

The answers to these questions, I believe, are in a culture that encourages girls restrict their eating in an unhealthy way. But there's also been a decided change in the kinds of foods young people eat.

A recent study showed that the median intake of girls ages 11 to 19 provided only 51 to 67 percent of the Recommended Daily Dietary Allowance of calcium, iron, vitamin A, magnesium, zinc, copper and other critical nutrients, and about 80 to 90 percent of recommended calories.

That means half the girls in the United States are eating less than this. Healthy foods fuel growing brains and bones as well as strong bodies, but these girls aren't getting even the calories they need for healthy growth and development. They are severely undernourished.

Will these girls develop into well-rounded, capable, healthy adults? Or will they face a lifetime of health problems, like osteoporosis because they kept vital nutrients from their bodies? Will they have financial troubles because they were too weak to learn in school and develop careers? I think the odds for future health problems are frightening.

The documentation for this appalling news is in the Third Report on Nutrition Monitoring, published in two large volumes by the U.S. Department of Health and Human Services and the U.S. Department of Agriculture at the end of 1995. It brings together information on nutrition from surveys, analyses and monitoring systems.[1]

Adequate diets

Children start out eating in healthy ways. Until age 11, most girls eat well-balanced diets, with adequate calcium and iron, except they tend to be lower in calories — 1,753 calories, only 73 percent of the RDA of 2,400. Boys, too, seem to be adequate at all ages in both nutrients and calories. They're even eating slightly less fat than kids did 10 years ago.

The Bogalusa Heart Study of children in the American South documents these trends. Children start out eating healthy diets, but as they reach adolescence, their diets change. As teens, the number increases of kids eating only two-thirds of recommended nutrients. They foods they eat also change toward the high-calorie, low-nutrient foods, more dessert and snack foods.

Even though the children currently in the study are heavier than kids studied 14 years ago, they eat fewer calories and less fat and cholesterol. Other studies show the same thing. But it's not clear if today's children are that much more sedentary or if diet changes may be causing new problems in overweight.

What are kids eating?

Young people today are eating twice as much crackers, popcorn, pretzels and corn chips. More grain-based foods. More pasta with sauce, rice dishes, tacos, burritos — and pizza, the all time favorite. Three times as much soda pop. More desserts and candy.[2]

What's missing? They eat less meat, eggs, milk, fruit and vegetables.

One in two teenagers drinks no milk, compared with three out of four who were milk drinkers in the 1970s. Those children who do drink milk just drink about 1 1/2 to two cups a day, not the recommended 3 cups. Few eat the recommended five daily servings of fruits and vegetables, except for younger children.

The favorite vegetable: Potatoes, (especially french fries and potato chips), followed by tomato dishes. Low on the list: green beans, corn, green peas, lima beans, and the nutrient-packed dark greens or deep-yellow vegetables that people are encouraged to eat regularly.

Cave man diet

An odd thing about this kind of diet, it's almost full circle from what our ancestors ate. Early humans ate a diet high in meat, and lots of fruits and vegetables. It was focused on these three food groups (after weaning from mother's milk at age 4 or 5). They ate almost no grain, according to anthropologists.

In Europe those early meat-eaters 30,000 years ago were tall and strong with sound bones. They grew six inches taller than their descendents who settled down to farming, raised grains, vegetables and

Figure 1

Median daily nutrient intake

Percentage of 1989 recommended values (RDA)[1]

	Female						Male					
	12-15 years			16-19 years			12-15 years			16-19 years		
	White	Black	Mex/Am	White	Black	Mex/Am	White	Black	Mex/Am	White	Black	Mex/Am
Calcium	62	51	66	66	52	56	90	60	85	103	76	79
Iron	67	65	68	63	69	68	128	110	119	146	119	114
Copper	67	62	59	63	66	67	81	76	79	93	87	84
Vitamin A	63	64	59	73	60	54	85	55	70	77	55	67
Magnesium	64	70	74	62	58	66	103	85	97	78	68	70
Zinc	67	71	72	70	78	72	77	59	70	90	82	80
Vitamin E	70	85	63	72	78	76	68	74	67	93	92	77
Phosphorus	87	81	94	88	87	90	118	97	114	141	126	122
Vitamin B$_6$	78	96	83	75	83	87	110	92	95	104	93	83

HHS, NHANES III, 1988-91/AFRAID TO EAT 1997

fruit, and almost no meat. And it took those descendants until the Industrial Revolution on a diet that again included plenty of meat, eggs and milk, to gain back that six inches in height.[3]

Today, nutritionists advise that a sound food plan contains balance, moderation and variety from five food groups — grains, fruits, vegetables, meat group, and milk group. These fill the food pyramid. And at the top is a small niche for fats and sweets, special foods to eat sparingly *(see Food Guide Pyramid).*

Now we are seeing our children again shift their diets, this time away from modern advice for five food groups, and even farther from that ancient diet of three groups, to focusing on a single group — a diet based almost entirely on grains: bread, pasta, cereals, baked goods, crackers. Plus, youngsters today are pulling down that small niche group of candy, desserts, high-fat snacks, soft drinks, and expanding it into a major part of their food intake.

This is a significant departure from five groups eaten in moderation, balance and variety — to basically only one without much variety. It's extremely limited. How can it be healthy? Why are parents allowing it? Can it be because many parents are also eating this way?

Some parents think they can fill a nutrition gap with pills and food supplements. But they are fooling themselves: real food is what counts in a healthy lifestyle.

For example, take phytochemicals, one of the hottest new areas in cancer research. It's estimated there may be over 100 different phytochemicals in just one serving of vegetables. And we haven't identified them all, much less which ones are most effective against cancer. Other nutrients and their roles are just starting to be discovered.

If you eat a pill instead of the vegetables, you lose out. This is why variety is so important in food choices, to ensure getting a wide variety of nutrients.

Iron and calcium

Two of the most critical nutrients for healthy growth and development are iron and calcium. Yet most teenage girls in the U.S. consume just two-thirds or less of what they need. *(Fig. 1 and 2:*

Note that intake values vary slightly between these two charts due to somewhat differing population data and analysis, even though basically the same report.)

Girls especially need iron because they lose iron-rich blood every month in menstruation. Iron carries oxygen through the blood to cells, helping to produce energy. Girls who are low in iron will feel fatigued weak, listless, irritable and have headaches. And they'll have a harder time learning.

The damage children may suffer from lack of iron may not be reversible. Iron-deficient children commonly have shortened attention span, lower intelligence scores, and reduced overall intellectual performance. Some studies find active iron therapy fails to improve mental performance for many anemic children.[4]

Iron isn't easily absorbed by the body. In fact, 90 percent is lost unless some heme iron from animal products is eaten. The body absorbs three times as much if the meal includes meat, so vegetarians need to plan carefully to compensate. Even a small amount of heme iron from meat, poultry, fish and eggs helps the body absorb iron. Vitamin C also helps iron absorption.

Calcium is important for every child to maximize bone develop-

---

Figure 2

Median daily nutrient intakes

percent of RDA

	Calories	Iron	Calcium	Vitamin A
Female				
12-15 years	82%	57%	57%	67%
16-19 years	85	57	62	68

Other nutrients far below recommended intake levels at the median for girls ages 12-19 are: Vitamin E, Vitamin B6, phosphorus, magnesium, zinc and copper.[2]

USHHS NHANES III, 1988-91 ADVANCE DATA, NCHS (Nov 1994)/AFRAID TO EAT 1997 ment, but it is even more critical for girls. They're building bone mass until about age 25. Girls who don't drink enough milk, and especially if they are thin and dieting, may be setting themselves up for a lifetime of fragile bones, fractures and osteoporosis. Osteoporosis (literally, "porous bones") can be painful and expensive. Women with severe cases can break their ribs sneezing, or break a leg or a hip by standing the wrong way. It can rob women of an independent and active life — and I fear that these thin, dieting teenagers will be those women at mid-life.

Perhaps if these girls went into nursing homes to visit the unfortunate women crumpled down into themselves, whose bones have given way, maybe they'd value the strong bones they could be building now. Why don't they drink milk? They fear milk is fattening.

Why don't they eat iron-rich meat and eggs? It's the same sad story. Their fear of fat (even though they could eat them with very little or no fat).

Iron and calcium are only two of several dozen nutrients often lacking in nutrient-poor and unbalanced diets like these. These deficiencies cause longterm health problems related to growth and development and mental problems such as depression, confusion, hysteria and psychosis.

Apathy in the press

After two years these statistics still have not been analyzed. I keep urging it, and health policy makers keep telling me, "the big concern now is obesity" so they'll be looking at that first. It's true obesity is an urgent concern; many youngsters are still eating too much of high-fat foods. But it seems to me starvation is even more urgent — some youngsters are dying now of starvation. They are not dying from obesity.

Yet when these figures came out in October 1994, they did not even hit the national press. Most experts are still unaware they exist.

In both the media and public health bureaucracy, there appears to be an overwhelming apathy toward the plight of adolescent girls. The attitude seems to be that dieting and losing weight is normal for girls, so deficiencies can be expected.

"We have become all too familiar with sociocultural studies supporting the fact that young women in our country are badly in need
of attention, that they are being cheated, invalidated, and robbed of
their voices," charges Paula Levine, PhD, an eating disorder specialist in Miami.[5]

Missing out on meat

Children and adolescents missing out on meat, as many are today, is a serious matter that needs to be addressed by pediatricians,
nutritionists and health policy makers.

It has become trendy and politically correct in the media and
certain health circles to denigrate the contribution of meat to the
American diet. This is not supported by mainstream nutrition.

Certainly vegetarianism can be healthy, but as being practiced by
young people today in the U.S., often it is not. Two radical fringe
groups are exerting tremendous pressure against eating meat: the
overzealous environmental groups which mistakenly believe all land
can be cropped and that grazing animals is a "waste" of land; and
radical animal rights groups determined to convert young people to
the vegan lifestyle, to eating no animal products at all. And they are
adept at enlisting the media.

In denouncing these radical animal rights groups, the American
Medical Association says, "The AMA continues to marvel at how
effectively a fringe organization of questionable repute continues to
hoodwink the media."[6]

This is a dangerous agenda that calls for investigation. There is
no evidence that eating lean red meat is unhealthy in any way, and
volumes of scientific evidence that meat is health-promoting, and
especially for children and youth.

But this trendy notion is having a profound impact on the health
of children.

From coast to coast, eating disorder specialists tell me they are
seeing many new vegetarians — young children with eating problems, stunted growth, fragile bones, and stress fractures, who are
responding to a frightening message brought by animal rights activists into their schools. They also see a second kind of new vegetarian

— girls with eating disorders who fear meat is fattening.

"This is very dangerous for kids," says William Jarvis, PhD, Loma Linda University, president of the National Council Against Health Fraud.

Patricia Hunt, a registered nurse in Mukilteo, Wash., whose daughter Jennifer became a vegan after an animal rights group came into her school, recently told the *Wall Street Journal* she was "angry with the schools and the propaganda."

Hunt says Jennifer refuses even to take vitamins prescribed by her doctor because they are made from animal products. "She has a hotline number that she calls before she'll take anything."

Parents from Maine to California complained in the *Journal* article about animal rights activists and the teachers who invited them into the classroom to push the vegan lifestyle. No longer able to influence their children's healthy eating, these parents were further frustrated by being harangued about cooking ingredients, compelled to fix two sets of meals, and lectured about their own eating.

"There is a sense that these kids have been traumatized . . . influenced by the message that the animal rights people are taking into the schools. When children see these gory pictures about mistreated animals, they really don't have the ability to stop and say 'Wait a minute, is there another side to this story?'" explains Monika Woolsey, MS, RD, Nutrition Consultant and Eating Disorders Specialist in Arizona.

She says vegetarianism seems to be a politically correct way to have an eating disorder. "Many of these children have suffered from emotional, physical or sexual abuse or trauma, and it's almost as if they've made a vow not to hurt animals as they have been hurt."

They struggle with self worth, says Woolsey. "They believe their self-esteem comes from what they do, not who they are, and part of what they do is eat. So they are trying to eat perfectly, and they get this black and white sense of what is perfect: 'If I'm a nice person I'll be a vegetarian, and if I'm not a nice person I'll eat meat.' That's how black and white their thinking gets when you talk to them."

In Kentucky, dietitians have successfully launched an educational campaign to inform educators and parents about this threat of animal rights misinformation and deception targeted to their schools.

Nancy Tullis, RD, chair of the Reliable Nutrition Information section of the Louisville Dietetic Association, says, "Self appointed 'nutritionists' should not be allowed to go into the schools to present an emotional diatribe about society's shortcomings in the areas of nutrition, air, soil, water and animal cruelty, place blame on certain groups, and then irresponsibly teach the new vegan diet pattern, leaving some inadequate brochures behind. The children will go home short on facts and long on anger. We do not believe in setting children up for this emotional confrontation with their families."

Cutting fat

In the past decade, both children and adults have reduced fat from 36 to 34 percent of total calories, bringing them closer to the goal of 30 percent or less set by the Dietary Guidelines for Americans.

High fat intake is known to contribute to obesity, and is a risk factor for chronic disease. Fat that is eaten is easily converted to fat in the cells, unlike carbohydrate which burns up one-fourth of the calories in conversion and protein, of which little if any is stored as fat. Before discovering this and its link to chronic disease, Americans were eating an average of 41 to 42 percent fat — plus some 25 percent in sugars, leaving only about one-third of calories for more nutritious food choices.

Many youngsters still eat a lot of fat. However, some professionals debate whether dropping fat to 30 percent is too low for children.

Lowfat diets are not appropriate for children or the elderly, insists Alfred Harper, PhD, professor emeritus of biochemistry at the University of Wisconsin.

Harper faults the Dietary Guidelines because they are being applied to children. "These guidelines represent a sharp change in direction in health policy and dietary guidance, away from dietary advice to ensure that growth and development of children will not be impaired — and toward a program of dietetic medicine to prevent chronic and degenerative diseases," he told attendees at the 1996 Southern California Food Industry Conference in Costa Mesa, Calif.

Harper said the assumption that limiting fat intake in children will provide them with healthier lives as adults has not been validated by research. He also questions why the current drop in fat has not been accompanied by a decrease in overweight, as expected, but rather by a sharp increase. While others suggest this must stem from further inactivity, Harper argues that lowfat foods may be making people fatter, because they lose satiety cues they have come to rely on. Perhaps they do not feel as satisfied with the foods they are eating today, often processed and prepackaged, as when eating home-cooked foods in family meals at home.

And nutritionists are well aware that the emphasis on reducing fat has backfired in some cases, causing many youth to develop fat phobias and reduce their fat intake to dangerously low levels. A downside of the new nutrition labels is that they make it easier to select foods with zero fat.

This is painfully apparent in working with women on college campuses. Cynthia De Tota, MA, RD, University Nutritionist at Syracuse University in New York, tells me that college girls' obsession with thinness and dieting is excruciating. Fat has become an evil.

At one sorority, girls who ate any food containing fat during rush week were required to pay into a penalty pot. In a drama group, students told her the newest trend is if a food has any fat "you can eat, but don't swallow — spit it out."

Girls in campus cafeterias typically choose a meal of only a lettuce salad with nonfat dressing and a Diet Coke. Many have taken up smoking to control weight.

"It's such a frustrating problem, because when I start talking about the dangers of over-restricting fat, these young women don't seem to value their health enough to make any changes. The value they place on physical appearance and body weight outweighs the value they place on their health.

"I have analyzed some students' fat intakes to be only 4 percent of their needs. When I give them the results, they are proud instead of concerned. They have an intense fear of fat. They really think if they increase their fat intake, they'll immediately gain weight.

"I encourage them to try a small change just for a week, anything else is overwhelming: 'If you could add one or two tablespoons of peanut butter on your bagels at breakfast. Just try it for a week and see if it makes a difference in how you feel.' Some will do it, and they say they feel so much better, are more alert, and don't fall asleep in class. But many are afraid to try."

Teenage girls who are eating in the recommended range of about 2,000 calories, balanced with physical activity, can meet the recommended 30 percent fat with about 600 calories in fat, or 67 grams. This means averaging a comfortable 22 grams at each of three meals. It's a long way from zero fat.

Skipping breakfast

Dieting teens commonly skip breakfast. So do adults.

But recent studies confirm starting the day without breakfast affects thinking, problem solving, verbal fluency, ability to recall and use newly acquired information, attention span, and educational achievement. Breakfast is especially needed by youngsters who are nutritionally at-risk, or are dieting, one study shows.

Children ages 9 to 11 who ate breakfast were faster and more accurate in school and had better memories. Iron deficiencies, anemia, and other nutrition deficiencies found to be highly prevalent in these youth strongly affected their thinking ability. Schools that provided breakfast found that kids were more likely to come to school and perform better in the classroom.[7]

Kids are also eating more food outside the home. One-third of students get nearly half their calories away from home, up considerably from the 1970s. This probably also contributes to their unbalanced food choices. Teenage boys report eating most often at fast food restaurants rather than the school cafeteria.[8]

Confusing the public

Often it's the lifestyle choices families make that mean the difference between whether their children develop weight and eating problems or not.

We need to return to the principles of moderation, balance and variety. These are the key factors in healthy food choices, and we can use them as a key to many other positive lifestyle choices, as well.

But it seems that Americans have a habit of going to extremes. If fat tastes good, then overeat; if it adds pounds, opt for "zero" fat. On the one hand people feel recklessly indulged, on the other, sensuously virtuous.

Can we find peace instead with the simplicity of moderation and balance, and let this misplaced "excitement" flow into other areas of our lives?

One of the biggest problems affecting nutrition at this time is the confusion in the media about foods and health. Instead of clear messages of health, they are of contradiction, risk and scare-mongering, "good foods, bad foods."

Parents are confused and fearful over the many supposed risks they read about daily in the headlines of their newspapers. Children reflect this confusion and fear.

The problem is, in this time of instant communication, we get an overload of unimportant information. Newspapers cannot resist featuring the health terrorist of the day. The public gets startling news, here today and forgotten tomorrow, but is left shaken, a bit more fearful.

On a recent flight from Chicago, where I did a stint on the Oprah Winfrey Show, I sat next to a Kentucky businessman who traveled often.

"I was on a plane the morning that headlines read, 'coffee raises cholesterol,'" he told me. "No one drank coffee. On another flight the newspaper said coffee prevents suicide, and everyone was calling for coffee. Another time it was orange juice, and everyone drank orange juice. We're crazy, aren't we?"

Right. And headlines sell papers. Nevertheless, the media needs to be more responsible in helping people put these bits of information in perspective.

Sources used may be barely credible. There are headline-grabbing, irresponsible researchers. Experts today are often embarrassed and chagrined by "health terrorist" messages beamed out by two entities who know better: the Center for Science in the Public Interest, that stayed a million hands in mid-reach for movie popcorn and

Chinese takeouts, and the "Harvard group," with its never-ending, often-inappropriately reported Nurse's Study.

Harper regrets the trend toward categorizing foods as either good or bad, as medicines or health hazards.

It's important to restore confidence in the basic principle that health depends on the total diet, he says, not on a few special components. "This is of particular concern with the diets of children."

Harper also argues that blaming fat for the increase in chronic disease is a myth. This increase is a natural consequence of an aging population, he points out. Most people no longer die early of acute tragic causes. Most die in old age of chronic disease — and that's as it should be, he suggests.

Measures of despair

Eating well and living healthily contributes to feeling good about yourself. If suicidal thoughts and plans are an indication of how our youngsters are faring, they are not doing well. Girls especially are in trouble.

Nearly one-fourth of high school students nationwide reported they had seriously considered attempting suicide during the 12 months before the 1995 Youth Risk Behavior survey, a slight increase over 1993 (fig. 3).

But the rates are twice as high among girls, and highest among Hispanic girls. Of Hispanic girls, 34 percent reported seriously considering suicide, 26 percent made a suicide plan, 21 percent attempted suicide, and 7 percent had a suicide attempt that required medical attention, all during the 12 months preceding the survey. These are the highest rates of all. For white girls these figures are 32, 22, 10, 3 percent; for black girls, 22, 16, 11, 4 percent.

For boys the rates are: white, 19, 15, 5, 2; black, 17, 13, 7, 3; and Hispanic, 16, 13, 6, 3.

Girls were more likely to have considered, planned or attempted suicide when they were younger, as freshmen or sophomores. But this trend was somewhat reversed for boys.

What's going on with these girls? What part might malnutrition-induced low moods and depression play? What about their struggle with body image and low self esteem? What's happening to Hispanic girls? We need to know this to bring about healthy change.

Physical activity

Moderation, balance and variety make good sense for physical activity, too.

Children are the most active and physically fit of all Americans, averaging one to two hours of moderate or vigorous physical activity each day. But they're less active than their parents were as children — and they're developing habits that could turn them into inactive, overweight, unhealthy adults.

Most grow less active each year. Girls, especially, drop into sedentary lifestyles by age 15 or 16.

Researchers see a relationship between the widespread decrease in physical activity and the increasing prevalence of obesity, even though it's difficult to measure both physical activity and its relation to obesity in children.

What is clear, is that both children and adults live less active lives than their peers a few decades ago. Many people have changed their lifestyles in response to violence or feelings that they're unsafe. More

---

Figure 3

Suicide thoughts and behavior
percent of U.S. high school students[3]

	Thought seriously about attempting suicide*	Made a suicide plan*	Attempted suicide one or more times*
Female	30%	21%	12%
Male	18	14	6

*During the 12 months preceding the survey.

U.S. YOUTH RISK BEHAVIOR SURVEY 1995

parents work longer hours. There are more TV channels, more computer games, more video movies to watch, and the Internet to surf.

Children become less active with age

Boys are more active than girls, and the gap widens through high school and college, says researcher James Sallis, PhD, of San Diego State University. He reviewed six self-reported studies that included 33,238 boys and 32,902 girls ages 8 to 16.

He also looked at studies which measured their heart rates and actual physical activity. He found that boys and girls think they are more active than they actually are.

Still, boys ages of 6 to 17 are consistently about 15 to 25 percent more physically active than girls. Girls reduce their physical activity levels with age more than boys; their rate of decline is about two and a half times greater. Thus the gender gap widens with age. Girls may be at higher risk of activity-related health problems due to their more sedentary lifestyles, warns Sallis.

Further, he says this evidence suggests the need for reevaluating the reasons why girls are less fit than boys. It has been thought that gender differences in fitness were related to higher body fat for maturing girls, their lower muscle mass and hemoglobin concentrations.

But maybe that's not the major reason. Maybe this relatively new data on gender differences in physical activity is suggesting that the continuous decline in aerobic power for girls is related to the corresponding decline in activity. He urges that these gender differences be explored further.

Sallis also warns that more effective programs for preventing this decline need to be widely implemented.

Lifetime skills in PE class

The reputation of physical education class was never stellar. Now, despite many improvements, research shows that in many classes, students spend more time standing in line or watching others perform than being active themselves.

While most people agree that exercise is good for kids, they rarely follow through with efforts to motivate children or adequately train teachers, says Sallis, who has spent five years designing and researching a curriculum that makes physical education fun and engages a greater number of students, funded by the National Heart, Lung and Blood Institute.

"Kids spend 80 percent of their time standing around, and the majority get eliminated from many of the team sports," says Sallis.4

One study found the typical 40-minute physical education class provided youngsters with an average of less than 3 minutes of vigorous activity. The remainder of the class period was spent waiting in line, giving instructions and paper work.[9]

"It appears that a major opportunity to influence favorable physical activity in the United States is being missed in schools," says one Public Health report. The report points out that physical education classes seem to have little effect on the students' fitness levels or on increasing their lifelong physical activity.[10]

Physical education classes are further criticized for what they teach. Games and competitive sports, rather than lifetime activities, are the major part of existing programs. Federal researchers point out that for physical education classes to contribute to the health goal of lifelong activity, they should include moderate-intensity activities and should not focus exclusively on team-oriented sports activities.

The 1985 Children and Youth Fitness Study found that less than half of the PE curriculum was based on lifetime activities, which are the ones more readily carried into adulthood. These generally need only one or two people, such as bicycling, swimming and jogging, dancing and racquet sports. Competitive group and children's group games are not counted as lifetime activities.[11]

Despite their criticisms of how physical education is often taught, most researchers urge higher enrollments in daily PE classes at all age levels. Less than half of U.S. students now receive daily physical education, and Healthy People 2000 aims to increase this to at least 75 percent.[12]

Less fit are neglected

Nonathletic and less fit youngsters are the ones who need PE the most. Yet they are most neglected. One of every six children in the U.S. is so weak or uncoordinated as to be considered physically underdeveloped by the President's Council on Physical Fitness and Sports.

"That cold statistic barely hints at the personal trauma and social problems behind it. Such a child is likely to become a sedentary, overweight adult with all of the added health risks those conditions entail," says the Council.

Most schools still emphasize competitive sports, ball-handling skills, winning games, and court the best athletes. It's a system with little but humiliation to offer the unathletic or overweight child.

It's time to focus more effort on identifying and helping physically underdeveloped children, says the President's Council. This is "the most urgent task facing physical education and other youth activity programs."

The Council urges schools to test for fitness, as they do for reading and math, and enact remedial programs for students who don't meet standards. A special class is recommended, or if this is impractical, a separate exercise program for part of the session or the entire class participating in activities needed by the underdeveloped.

Most of these kids can achieve appropriate levels of physical fitness, say these experts. Teachers and parents need to understand the importance of fitness for each child in healthy growth, academic performance and prevention of weight problems.[13]

Girls discouraged from sports

Girls also tend to be neglected in physical education. They get far less encouragement to go into organized sports than boys. Often they are actively discouraged by family, friends, the institutions in charge of sports and health, and by what they see in the media.

More girls participate in sports than ever before, yet experts say they have a long way to go before they are treated equally.

Historically, women's sports were thriving during the 1920s and 1930s, and most high schools had girls' basketball teams, even though they were not always allowed to travel to other schools. But the end of the second world war brought a change in the public mood and an end to much of this.

Girl's high school basketball teams were discontinued throughout most of the U.S. for 25 or 30 years beginning in the late 1940s.

In the era of "the feminine mystique" which ensued, vigorous sports were deemed too strenuous for girls. The national mood in those post war years turned toward encouragement of femininity and greater protectionism for girls. The feeling was that being on active sports teams could have harmful health and social effects for young women.

Iowa was one of the few states to continue girls' basketball through this period, claiming, against all odds, that exercise was healthy for girls. Ironically, new brain research suggests that exercise is important not only for health, but even in the development of intelligence. It shows that use of the large muscles in physical activity during adolescence is helpful in increasing nerve connections for higher brain development.

Girls basketball was reinstated in most high schools during the late 1960s and early 1970s. Title IX brought more equality for girls into athletics, and put pressure on school administrations to provide more sports for girls.

Yet the teens are a time when girls drop out of sports. Considerable evidence shows that their self-esteem drops, too, at this same time.

Melpomene, a Minneapolis-based women's sports research organization, is asking why this happens and how girls can be helped to continue their interest in sports after adolescence.

A recent Melpomene study finds younger girls, age 9 to 12, enjoy sports and describe them as a way they feel good about themselves. But older girls, age 12 to 17, while agreeing that they enjoy sports, cite major obstacles to being in sports. Among these are the behavior of boys and systems that favor male athletes.

These girls said boys in mixed groups often control games. Typical comments were:

"Boys, they like to hog the basketball."

"Even if you're right there, they won't pass the ball."

"In soccer we have half the girls standing out most of the time because all the boys are playing."

This male control was also evident in picking teams. The girls said boys were chosen first, and girls last: "Girls are always last."

Some girls said they hesitate to play on these mixed teams for fear of male criticism or of making a mistake. The girls also described a system in which boys and young men have more team choices, better equipment, and are taken more seriously by school and fans.

"At boys' games the whole stands are filled . . . (for girls' games) basically the parents are there."

"They get better coaches, more time, more fields to play."

The researchers were concerned that the teenage girls often prefaced their remarks with "I don't know."

The girls often said this before giving an opinion or fact, such as, "I don't know, I just love sports."

They cite research which shows girls enter adolescence full of confidence and sure of what they know, but three years later are unsure of themselves, and their knowledge becomes private.

Using the qualifier "I don't know" was seen as a way the girls protected themselves from criticism. In one focus group this qualifier was used almost 50 times to preface the girls' opinions. More use seemed linked to lower levels of self-esteem, confidence and competence, the researchers report.[8]

Youth Risk Behavior survey

Yet the outlook has improved greatly in the last decade. And the 1996 Olympics were an inspiration to female athletes.

The 1995 Youth Risk Behavior Survey shows schools are doing a better job and more youngsters are active at recommended levels. We're close to meeting the Healthy People 2000 objective in which 75 percent of children ages 6 to 17 will exercise 20 minutes three or more days per week.

The Youth Risk survey found that 64 percent of students (53 percent of black, 57 percent of Hispanic, and 67 percent of white students) in grades 9 to 12 meet the recommended criteria and 52 percent of girls compared with 74 percent of boys. These percentages are double the 1990 figures, but represent a slight drop from 1993.

This is at the modest level of vigorous activity for at least 20 minutes 3 days a week, which is a start.

Older students are still less active than younger ones. Girls show a steep drop in activity at this level from their freshman year to their senior year — from 62 percent who are active as freshmen to 42 percent. However, this drop was greater in 1990, from 31 percent down to 17 percent. Boys also dropped from their freshman to their senior year (80 to 67 percent).

The survey found that 60 percent of high school students were enrolled in PE classes, but only about one quarter attended classes daily. In an average PE class, 45 percent of the students spend at least 20 minutes exercising.

Half of all students play on at least one school sports team, with girls almost as likely to play on these teams as boys (42 vs 58 percent). But boys are much more likely to play on sports teams outside of school — 46 percent compared with 27 percent of girls.

During the month before the survey, 64 percent of girls said they exercised to lose weight or keep from gaining weight. So did 39 percent of boys.

News stories

Despite the encouraging example of the Olympics, girls have fewer women role models to look up to in athletics. Media coverage often ignores women's teams and women athletes.

When the media does focus on women in sports, it is often in a conflicting and confusing way that sends mixed messages to young girls. Women athletes are frequently portrayed in ways that emphasize their femininity, rather than their athletic skill and excellence in their chosen sport. This can cause much ambivalence for girls, uncertain whether their role is primarily one of athletic skill or personal appearance on the playing field.

Amy Terhaar Woodcock, a graduate student in sports management at the University of Minnesota, explains that the media has tried to find a way for female athletes to continue to fit into our culture's feminine ideals by pointing out that women are too frail for contact sports. Thus, reporters and cameras watch for female weaknesses and then exploit them through photos and stories.

She cites references which document how the media focuses on "sex specific rather than sport specific conditions or injuries" for women but not men. An injury which to a male athlete is attributed to the sport, is for a female athlete blamed on female weakness.

Sports magazines such as *Sports Illustrated,* avidly read each week by sports-minded girls and women as well as men, typically devote more space to swimsuit editions, pinup calendars and cheer-leaders at football games than to women athletes.

One study of *Sports Illustrated* covers from 1957 to 1989 found a decline in the number of times women were featured in active poses over these 22 years. Men were featured on the cover 782 times, and women 55 times. But of these 55 covers, only two showed women in active poses.

Another recent study examined pictures of female Olympic athletes and found they were often suggestive, emotional, or the women were shown away from their sport. Many focused on the female athlete's body in sexually suggestive ways. Emotional shots showed the athlete crying and being comforted by male coaches and family. Most of the photo captions mentioned feminine characteristics and often that the woman was short, rather than pointing out her athletic skill and achievements.

Women's sports are vastly under-represented in television, newspaper and sports magazines. A look at four daily newspapers found that women were the subjects of only 3.5 percent of all sports articles, and men, 81 percent. Men were pictured in 92 percent of all sports. Another study showed men's professional golf was shown 70 times on national television in 1993, while women's golf appeared only 13 times.

Woodcock studied the daily newspaper coverage of girls' and boys' high school ice hockey in the Twin Cities area in 1994-1995.

She found there were 65 boys teams and 24 girls teams in the Metropolitan area, but 89 percent of the newspaper space was devoted to boys' hockey, compared with 11 percent for girls' hockey. Articles on boys which had photos averaged 43 inches of print. Articles on girls with photos were much shorter, averaging 11 inches of print. The boys' stories had an average of one more photo per story and these were often action shots. Of the 35 photos of girls' high school hockey she found, only four showed the girls playing hockey.

When a female hockey player was chosen athlete of the week, she was pictured sitting on a bench holding her stick and gloves. An article headlined, "Small Stature, Big Talent," showed a photo that emphasized the girl's small size by cutting off her teammates' heads. The article referred to her as the "tournament darling." In a more positive portrayal, another newspaper featured the same athlete by focusing on her athletic talent, mentioning her size once, and running a photo that showed her on the ice, in uniform, shooting a puck.

This unequal newspaper, television and sports magazine coverage is reflected in sports books — even picture books for very young children.

A Melpomene Institute study found that even today girls are portrayed only about half as often as boys in picture books on sports which are aimed at children under grade two. Often girls are shown watching boys in action.

These are major improvements however. During the 1950s and 1960s, no girls at all were shown in this sample of books. The researchers looked at 105 books from the last 40 years containing 23 popular sports sampled from the sports category of the children's picture book directory *A to Zoo.*

Overall, nearly three times as many books from the last four decades had males as the only or major characters compared with females (58 percent to 20 percent). Males were identified as the only characters four times as often as females. Gender equality was portrayed in 17 percent of the books.[14]

Exercise excesses

While encouraging activity, we need to be aware of its abuses, too. Obsessive exercise can take over youngsters' lives.

Female athletes often engage in compulsive exercise to lose weight. For males there is a new emphasis on body sculpting and muscle building, which can become obsessive.

Karin Kratina, MA, RD, an exercise physiologist, dietitian and clinical outreach coordinator at the Renfrew Center in Florida, describes a typical scenario of a young woman with exercise dependence.

"She rises each morning at 5:30, hits the pavement for a brisk three miles, rain or shine, works out 45 minutes at the fitness center on lunch break, and goes to another health club after work for an hour of aerobics, half an hour on the Stairmaster and a half hour on the Lifecycle. She appears to be a motivated, fit and happy person but her legs ache constantly, as she continues to work out despite shin splints. When she stops for a time her depression and anxiety become so overwhelming, she can't wait to get back to her workouts."[15]

Obsessive exercise aimed at weight loss is often regarded as a secondary dependency to an eating disorder.

It's very common. Kratina suggests that at least half of anorexics and bulimics she is seeing probably deal with some form of exercise dependency.

"Stress injuries are common, and frequently the person exercises right through an injury so it can't heal properly," she says.

Menstrual dysfunction and amenorrhea are common among female athletes in a wide range of sports, and severe weight restrictions may be a major reason. These disturbances are associated with scoliosis and stress fractures in young ballet dancers. Delayed menarche, as late as age 19 or 20 for very thin female athletes and ballet dancers, is linked to osteoporosis and bone fractures, usually linked with a restrictive diet. (A somewhat delayed puberty, associated with thinness and higher activity levels at age 10 to 14, may be beneficial in reducing teenage pregnancy and reproductive cancer risk.)[16]

The "female-athlete triad" which includes eating disorders, amenorrhea and osteoporosis, is becoming well known among elite women athletes.

Struggling to be the best at a sport and at the same time coping with body changes is especially difficult for adolescent girls, because of societal pressures that promote thinness and beauty. Trying to control weight while focusing on training and performance may lead to a sense of frustration, guilt, despair and failure, and to a pattern of unhealthy eating and eating disorders.

Competing or training while dehydrated is an extremely hazardous practice which can inhibit sweating, and increase risk of temperature problems and heat stroke. This is a serious risk for wrestlers who dehydrate themselves for a day or more to lose weight for a match.

Severely restricting food and fluid can affect metabolism, body composition, performance and overall health. Fluid losses and resulting electrolyte disturbances can increase risk of cardiac arrhythmias, renal damage, impaired performance and increased chance of injury, say Garner and Rosen.[17] This also can affect heart output and body temperature. Concerns have also been raised about possible delayed growth and development during a period of active growth, and initiation of eating disorders.

Body fat dangerously low

The average young man, with normally about 14 to 16 percent body fat, will likely strive for 5 to 7 percent if he is serious about sports in which leanness can be a factor, says the U.S. Olympic Committee's Division of Sport Medicine and Science.

Many young female athletes also strive for 5 to 7 percent body fat, even though they might normally have body fat of 20 to 22 percent. The lowest safe minimum is often considered to be 5 percent for either boys or girls, and since measurements are notoriously inaccurate, there's much risk when readings are this low.

Severe dieting affects both the mind and body, but young athletes may not realize this. Garner and Rosen say young athletes may fear that the symptoms they experience — poor concentration, moodiness, irritability, anger, depression, feelings of inadequacy, anxiety, obsessional thinking, poor decision making and social withdrawal — are signs of deeper emotional disturbances.

"Skinny kid in a daze"

In calling for all states to raise body fat requirements for wrestlers from 5 to 7 percent, Charles Tipton, PhD, writing in the *Phy-*

sician and Sports Medicine, cites a study of elite high school wrestlers at the Iowa State Wrestling Championships which found 30 percent had only 5 percent or less body fat.

There is overwhelming evidence, Tipton says, that calorie restriction will ultimately diminish muscle strength. While student wrestlers need at least 1,500 to 2,200 calories per day, he says, they often eat between zero and 500 calories on days before a match.

My two sons, Rick and Mike, both high school wrestlers in the lower weights, were dedicated wrestlers, champions many times, so I understand this well. Often I felt helpless in aching for their good health against their determination to "make weight."

Discussing the medical aspects of wrestling, four specialists in wrestling research cited in the report express a strong concern for the abuses seen in the sport of wrestling. One warns that a sign of a wrestler losing too much weight is his loss of concentration — "a skinny kid walking around in a daze."

Another cites a study that found 7 percent of wrestlers use vomiting on a monthly basis, and 1 to 3 percent have used diuretics or laxatives.

The loss of three or four pounds is a big loss for the smaller wrestler, compared with the same amount for a 180-pounder, but it is often treated as the same by the coach.

The error factor of 5 to 7 percent, in even the best methods of testing body fat, is seen as a real problem, especially for the 103-pound wrestler.

More accurate testing of body fat, and dehydration through urine tests is suggested. More extensive use of certified athletic trainers and nutritionists, to minimize the negative effects of weight-cutting, is also needed.

Making weight

A Pennsylvania study of 368 high school wrestlers found that 42 percent had lost 11 to 20 pounds at least once in their lives. One-fourth were losing 6 to 10 pounds every week. After a match 30 to 40 percent reported being preoccupied with food and eating out of control. The wrestlers used a variety of aggressive methods to lose weight, including dehydration, food restriction, fasting, vomiting, laxatives and diuretics. "Making weight" was associated with fatigue, anger and anxiety.

Weight loss methods of college wrestlers were investigated with 42 college wrestlers by Suzanne Nelson Steen, MS, RD, and Shortie McKinney, PhD, RD.

Most were using the techniques of reducing and depriving food, dehydration, and strenuous exercise in daily training sessions.

During the season 37 percent of wrestlers did not meet the recommended dietary allowance (RDA) for calories. This is more severe, it is pointed out, because RDA does not account for their strenuous training activity. One-fourth did not meet two thirds of the criteria for vitamin C, iron, and thiamine, half did not meet it for vitamin A, and more than half for vitamin B6, magnesium, and zinc. Diets tended to be higher in fat and lower in carbohydrate than recommended.

Intake was extremely variable. For example, one 118 pound wrestler consumed 334 calories the day before the match, 4,214 calories in the evening after his match, and 5,235 the next day. His weekly loss and regain were each 12 pounds.

Food and fluid intake was typically minimal and sometimes zero for both days previous to the match.

In the allotted five hours between weigh-in and match, fluid and food were increased in an attempt to rehydrate and restore strength, but the researchers say this is insufficient time for restoring electrolyte balance or replenishing muscle glycogen concentration. They suggest that many wrestlers compete with greatly reduced carbohydrate stores, leading to premature fatigue and poor performance.

Among the wrestlers' nutrition misconceptions was the common view that starchy carbohydrates are fattening. One third avoided breads, pasta and potatoes.

They reported cravings for sweets when dieting.

After the season, their fat intake was considerably higher than either preseason or midseason, suggesting that perhaps deprivation increased preference for fat. Nutrition was generally adequate before and after the season.

Athletic trainers say that rapid weight loss for wrestlers can cause kidney and heart strain, low blood volume, electrolyte imbalances, increased irritability, depression, an inability to concentrate, and an increased vulnerability to eating disorders.

Dehydration

A high percent of the wrestlers used dehydration techniques. These included saunas (51 percent), wrestling in a heated room (74 percent), wearing rubber or plastic suits while exercising (42 percent), and restricting drinking (58 percent). On one team 5 percent of the wrestlers used laxatives and diuretics, and 11 percent used vomiting to lose weight, all hazardous practices.

It is ironic, say Steen and McKinney, that 83 percent of the wrestlers correctly believed their sudden weight loss affected their performance. They cite research showing that after a 4 percent loss of body weight from dehydration, muscle endurance drops 31 percent for isometric and 29 percent for isotonic exercise. Even four hours after rehydration, endurance was as much as 21 percent below initial levels. Not only does dehydration impair muscle performance, but it is extremely dangerous.[18]

CHAPTER **8**

Struggling with weight loss

■

Dieting is a common form of dysfunctional eating and perhaps the most acceptable. That also makes it dangerous.

Most teenage girls, no matter what their weight, are trying to lose weight, as are a quarter of teenage boys. Some dieters are children as young as 8 and 9. And one of two adults diet.[1]

These alarming statistics raise many questions. Is this supposed to be normal? What is happening to these children as they restrict nutrition, and constantly lose and gain weight? What happens to their growth, their bones, their brains, their lives?

Being overweight may have health risks, but that doesn't mean weight loss lessens those risks. Dieting can be dangerous and uncertain, and its risks include injury and death from diet products, semistarvation, and weight loss itself.

Weight loss methods and dangers

Dieting — in all its forms — is big business, with a price tag of $30 to $50 billion annually in the U.S. alone. The thinness culture has created a need in people from childhood to old age and there are plenty who are trying to meet it — for a price.

Even the Food and Drug Administration is succumbing to the pressure. In April 1996 it approved a diet drug which had not been

A doctor's weight loss education
by Allen King, MD

For the past 20 years I have seen over 5,000 obese patients for weight reduction and weight related diseases. The results of my attempts to improve their disease state by weight loss were, at best, short-lived.

Initially, I thought obesity was caused by lack of knowledge. I gave patients an outline of the caloric content of foods. In a follow-up period of four weeks to four months, the average patient lost eight ounces. Half gained weight!

I next tried behavior modification and recruited a dietitian to provide a more individualized diet. In a three month follow up, the average patient lost only five pounds.

With the popular movement to liquid diets and their initial great success, I then tried a rigidly controlled program. Over 500 patients were placed on 500 to 1000 calorie diets with behavior modification. The average patient lost 50 pounds in six months. I felt we had finally succeeded. A three year follow up, however, uncovered an average 60 pound regain.

Certainly, I thought, what was needed was more control. Gastric surgeries were unacceptable due to the mortality and morbidity rate. Anorexic medications were of limited use. My two patients who elected jaw wiring lost weight initially, then regained. The Garren Gastric bubble seemed the ideal solution — a plastic balloon inflated in the stomach. Weight loss did occur, but only in patients who developed ulcers and bowel obstructions.

I then became disillusioned and found myself avoiding discussing diet approaches with patients. Each method was followed by failure, and worse, guilt on the patient's part for "failing."

I now realize it is not the doctor's role to control the patient. Responsibility for change is with the patient. Change takes time and progress is variable. I now tell patients it takes five years to change. Patients who are able to change benefit greatly from their increased self knowledge and self acceptance.[1]

Allen King is currently using a nondiet approach in treating diabetic patients, with Dana Armstrong, Registered Dietitian, in private practice in Salinas, Calif.

studied in patients for more than one year.

Losing weight can be so difficult that for most, dieting is not simply a matter of eating less and cutting fat. Dieters invest in restrictive diets, drugs, gimmicks, surgery, smoking and purging — methods which damage a person's body, mind and pocketbook.

If even one worked, would we have so many? I don't think so.

Here are some popular methods for reducing weight:

- Surgery: gastric bypass and others
- Liposuction, tummy tuck
- Jaw wiring, gastric balloon
- Very low calorie diet (400-800 calorie), liquid or "protein sparing"
- Low and moderately low calorie diets (1,000 calorie or above)
- Behavior modification
- Drugs and diet pills claimed to speed metabolism, suppress appetite and/or block digestion
- Laxatives
- diuretics
- Smoking
- Meal supplements
- Weight loss centers providing diet and various combinations of exercise, pills, products, wraps
- Weight loss support groups
- Hypnotism
- Body wraps
- Aroma therapy
- Spot reducers, creams and lotions
- Herbal weight loss teas
- Herbal treatments, detoxifying the body
- Acupuncture and acupressure devices, for ear, wrist or soles of the feet
- Passive exercise tables, electrical stimulators
- Exercise and exercise equipment
- Gum
- Chinese soap

These methods are being used by children and teens. Some are self-prescribed, some medically monitored. They may be administered by professionals, multi-disciplinary medical teams, lay leaders, self-proclaimed gurus, or con artists. Most often, the consumer, who may be as young as age 9, quietly picks her own diets and diet products.

Unfortunately, there is little evidence of longterm success by any of these methods and some are extremely high risk.

While these methods promise dramatic results, credible information about the safety and effectiveness of most diet products and programs is simply not available.[2]

C. Wayne Callaway, an associate clinical professor of medicine at George Washington University, testified at congressional hearings in 1990 as a physician and on behalf of the American Board of Nutrition.[3]

"With rare exceptions, none of the popular commercially available programs for treating obesity is based on current scientific knowledge." If they were, they could no longer promise rapid weight loss, he said.

The lack of properly trained professionals in the weight loss industry is also a concern. "Supervision of such programs varies from none, to instantly created certified counselors, to physicians with little or no training in this area, to a few physicians and registered dietitians and behavioral psychologists who truly have the required expertise," Callaway said.

Pediatric experts claim their successes. But it's nearly impossible to validate their claims since research shows that most kids who are overweight — 60 percent of overweight 7-year-olds — will outgrow it.

Why dieting rarely works

The simple answer to why dieting doesn't work is that your body doesn't want it to. The human body defends its normal weight through a highly regulated system. That weight was once called the "setpoint," a term that lost favor because it implied a weight set at birth.

But just as the body regulates salt in the blood stream and body temperature, it also tries to keep its normal weight. If a person eats more calories than usual, the body tries to burn them off. If a person eats fewer calories than needed, the body tries to save on energy.

That's why weight loss treatment and dieting don't work. In fact, it's why there are so many different methods to lose weight, because none of them really work. The faster a person loses weight, the more quickly it is restored. Nutritionists no longer believe in a simple numbers game, in which they count calories in and calories out to come up with pounds lost. It doesn't work over the long term, and anything less than long term is irrelevant.

But yes, there are successes.

I'm haunted by some of them — gaunt, hollow-eyed young women wholly focused on their day's allotment of food.

The real successes I'm seeing aim at improving lifestyle habits, helping people change gradually to living more actively, eating moderately, relieving stress, and letting weight come off naturally as a result. Weight stays off when lost this way, because both habit and "set point" are changed. For individuals willing to do this, it can be a healthy change.

Perhaps at some time scientists will develop effective drugs that work for most people and are safe from terrible side effects. But at this time? Not really. That "everyone" is taking the new diet pills, is no guarantee. My basic advice holds: Wait at least two years after your friends and colleagues become enthusiastic about any new way to lose weight; by then, you'll know. So far it's proved good advice.

Certainly, for children and teens, it seems wise to delay — they have time to wait, and many years to regret a wrong decision.

Who is trying to lose weight?

Almost everyone. Several recent surveys of students show similarly frightening results: Most girls diet. And a study of Cleveland teens found that seven out of 10 white girls, six in 10 black girls had lost at least five pounds on one of their dieting attempts, as had four in 10 white and black boys *(fig. 1)*.[4]

More than one third of these girls were currently dieting, including 40 percent of white girls and 38 percent of black girls.

These kids used some dangerous weight loss methods, including semi-starvation, vomiting, diet pills, laxatives and diuretics. One-third of the dieting girls, and one-fourth of dieting boys said they fasted for 24 hours at least once a week.

"This is very disturbing," said Laurie Humphries, PhD, director of the Eating Disorders Clinic, University of Kentucky. "Frequently, we find these adolescents come in, 5-foot-one and 100 pounds . . . and (say) they need to be 89 pounds."

"Our study confirms that high school students feel very pressured to shape their bodies into the popular mold, and that increasing percentages of both boys and girls are dieting and purging in an attempt to accomplish this," said Lillian Emmons, PhD, RD, the nutritional anthropologist at Cleveland State University who directed the study.

Figure 1

Dieting and purging

among high school students[2]

	Girls		Boys	
	White	Black	White	Black
Dieters	77%	61%	42%	41%
Liquid diet	14	24	6	9
Diet pills	23	16	6	0
Laxatives	7	18	5	2
Diuretics	5	11	1	2
Vomiting	16	3	7	0
Monthly or more often	8	1	–	–
Fasting monthly or more often	35	40	29	25

Percent of total

Dieting and inappropriate dieting behaviors are widely practiced by U.S. high school students. Total 1,269 students, Cleveland State University study.

HWJ/OBESITY & HEALTH NOV/DEC 1992/CDC

The high dieting rates she found among boys is much higher than earlier reports, and yet may be under-reported, says Emmons. Of particular concern, she suggests, are the 10 percent of male dieters who lost 10 pounds twice as often as any other group and 62 pounds or more through dieting.

Emmons says meaningful education on reasonable expectations for body shape and size, and the negative effects of dieting and purging on future health and weight maintenance need to be taught, beginning before the preadolescent growth spurt.

But this is not happening or, if it is, "not as powerful as other cultural pressures," she warns. "The amount of purging shown in this study is cause for concern because of the potentially damaging effects purging can have on health."

Young athletes in sports and performance arts that emphasize leanness are at a special risk for harmful attempts to control the size and shape of their bodies. These include gymnastics, wrestling, judo, boxing, weight lifting, bodybuilding, figure skating, diving, ballet, dance, horse racing and distance running.[5]

Vomiting and laxatives are commonly used by female college athletes in several sports, several studies have shown.[6] Many high school wrestlers use extreme fluid and food deprivation in their efforts to "make weight" for a match.

"If there's a way to lose weight, a wrestler will find it," said Don Herrmann, associate director of the Wisconsin Interscholastic Athletic Association. "I've seen self-induced vomiting, laxative abuse, excessive water and food deprivation, even a self-induced bloody nose."[7] Dehydration techniques include saunas (51 percent), wrestling in a heated room (74 percent), wearing rubber or plastic suits while exercising (42 percent), and restricting drinking (58 percent), in one study. Add to the list diuretics.[8]

Diet pill abuse

Diet pills are another popular, and harmful, dieting method, even being used by small children. One in three teens have tried them. In the Cleveland study white kids seemed to use diet pills more often than black kids, up to 23 percent of white girls compared to 16 percent of black girls.[9]

The only over-the-counter weight loss drug approved by the FDA is PPA (phenylpropanolamine). Pills containing PPA are readily available at any grocery, drug, chain or convenience store, under such names as Dexatrim, Accutrim, Control, Dex-A-Diet, Diadex and Prolamine. Many teenage girls confess they shoplift these off the shelves and take them by the box.

In addition to PPA pills are the many quack pills, illegally claiming they suppress appetite, speed up metabolism, block fat or calorie absorption, or otherwise alter body functions to bring about "safe, easy, fast" weight loss. Often sold as "natural" or "herbal," these products are usually labelled as food supplements to avoid being confiscated by FDA. The claims you saw in the advertisement or television infomercial are no where to be found on the label in the health food store.

Many of these kinds of pills have won our Slim Chance Awards, given each January for the "worst" weight loss products of the year by *Healthy Weight Journal* and the National Council Against Health Fraud. Weight loss fraud works for kids because they, like many adults, want to believe there are easy ways to lose weight. The quack exploits this with a mixture of mysticism, pseudoscience and sensationalism, says Burton Love, FDA Midwest Regional Director. Many authorities agree that there is more fraudulent and misleading information about nutrition and weight than there has ever been, and it is being marketed effectively with enormous profits, in high-tech, highly targeted ways.

There's an endless supply of "magical" items for weight loss. In the last 11 years I've reported on scores of questionable diet pills, and have stacks of advertisements awaiting review. And if these ads find me, they are finding our children, too.

Parents and health professionals have pleaded with the FDA and Congress to take diet pills containing PPA off the shelves and restrict them to prescription sales to adults.

Approved as a diet aid in 1979 (when it was believed effective), PPA is found in some cold medicines as well as diet pills. Over $40 million dollars are spent yearly on advertising PPA diet products.

Sales of PPA should be restricted for minors, said Vivian Meehan, president of the National Association of Anorexia Nervosa and Associated Disorders. She urged that diet pills, laxatives, diuretics and emetics be sold only under a doctor's prescription for those under age 18, and sold to adults from behind the pharmacy counter; never from an open shelf or near products identified as diet aids.

Young people do use these diet pills. In a survey of Michigan State University students, one in five said they'd started using PPA diet pills between age 12 and 16. Nearly half the women and 6 percent of the men had taken a PPA dietary drug; 27 percent of the women within the past 12 months; 3 percent in the past 24 hours. Even 9 percent of those who perceived themselves as slightly underweight had used PPA diet pills in the last 12 months.

None had ever consulted a physician about their use, even though labels advise this for users under age 18. Many took more than the recommended daily limit of 75 mg of PPA. About one-fourth of the women students using diet pills had also double-dosed, using other PPA-containing products at the same time. One young woman with a severe cold had taken a diet pill and four nonprescription decongestant products containing PPA within 24 hours of the interview — a total of 675 mg.

Daily use of appetite suppressant diet pills may cause a rebound effect of fatigue and hyperphagia, insomnia, mood changes, irritability and, in extremely large doses, psychosis, say Allan Kaplan and Paul Garfinkel in Medical issues and the Eating Disorders.[10] Even when used correctly, PPA can cause dangerous reactions. It leads all other major non-prescription drugs in the number of adverse drug reactions and in the number of contacts with Poison Control Centers, a total of nearly 47,000 in 1989.

Other side effects documented include fatal strokes, dangerously high blood pressure, heart rhythm abnormalities, heart muscle and kidney damage, hallucinations, seizures, psychosis, headaches, nervousness and insomnia, cerebral hemorrhage, higher intercerebral pressure, nausea, vomiting, anxiety, palpitations, reversible renal failure, disorientation, psychotic behavior and death.

Furthermore, PPA is regarded by most users as ineffective and no data at all contradicts this.

A bereaved father testified at the 1990 congressional subcommittee hearings on the weight loss industry, protesting the easy availability of diet pills at groceries, discount outlets and corner drug stores.

"The lights went out in our lives on July 12, 1989, when our beautiful, fun-loving, and soon-to-be-married daughter, Noelle, died of cardiac arrest. These stores have no more business selling these drugs to children than they do liquor to a minor."[11]

Ephedrine

In May 1995, the FDA warned consumers about ephedrine, a drug supposedly used to combat asthma or keep people awake. But it's become a popular diet drug, especially among kids.

In March 1994, 10 Texas teenagers were taken to emergency rooms after overdosing on ephedrine. After 37 hospitalizations and two suspected deaths, Texas Health Commissioner David Smith in May 1994, temporarily banned a popular diet supplement containing ephedrine, Formula One, and prohibited the sale of ephedrine products to young people under age 18, according to the special report *Weight Loss Quackery and Fads,* published by Healthy Weight Journal.[12]

The FDA warned consumers not to buy or ingest Nature's Nutrition Formula One products that contain both Ma huang (ephedrine) and kola nut.

Any overdose with ephedrine is extremely risky and can start the heart racing, cause heart palpations and death. Yet overdosing is common with diet pills.[13] In the past two years, the FDA reported over 800 adverse reactions to ephedrine-containing products including at least 17 deaths. Reactions included life-threatening conditions including irregular heartbeat, heart attack, angina, stroke, seizures, hepatitis and psychosis. Temporary conditions such as dizziness, headache, memory loss, and gastrointestinal distress were also reported.[14]

Amphetamines

In their youth, many of today's large people were prescribed amphetamines by their doctors, and have as a result struggled with amphetamine addiction.

Gloria, now 43, was prescribed her first diet pills at age 12. In the book *Real Women Don't Diet*, by Ken Mayer, she explains, "They weren't called 'yellow jackets' or 'uppers' back then. They were just some little yellow pills given to a physically healthy twelve-year-old to lose weight. Before my mother had taken me to the family doctor, I had spent many hours crying and feeling ashamed because I was always the biggest girl in the class . . . Withdrawing from years of diet pills, which meant having vivid hallucinations and periods of extreme paranoia and finally becoming bulimic, were the most dangerous, physically damaging aspects of my war with my body, but the psychological damage and pain have been far more lasting."[15]

For most children, the pills were just one of many other types of treatments, both medically administered and self-prescribed.

Marcia G. Hutchinson, now a psychologist and author of *Transforming Body Image*, recounts her experiences. "From a very early age, I was subjected to state-of-the-art diet methods — amphetamines at age six, a ten-day hospitalized water fast at fifteen, and a dizzying array of restrictive regimes in between. I grew up in the '40s and '50s, when dieting was not the household word it is today. I was the only person that I knew who was always either on a diet, failing at a diet, planning a diet, or rebounding from a diet . . . It was dieting, and not some intrinsic neurosis, that made me into a compulsive overeater. Therefore it was dieting, not compulsive overeating, from which I really needed to recover . . . I needed to learn to trust in my own ability to self-regulate, and give myself permission to eat with pleasure."[16]

Surgery

Gastric surgery is usually not advised for children under age 17. The 1991 Gastrointestinal Surgery Consensus Development Conference Panel did not recommend surgery for adolescents.4 Surgery is risky even for adults.

Yet children do die from it. A review of gastric surgeries at the University of Florida Department of Surgery, Gainesville, showed three deaths within the first year among 11 children who had jejunoileal bypasses. Three others had severe complications requiring reanastomosis.

Thirty-nine surgeries for weight loss had been performed on adolescents from age 11 to 19 at that institution during the past 11 years.[17]

About 15,000 people have weight-reduction surgeries each year. About 180, or 1.2 percent, are listed as being age 18 to 19.[18]

Summer weight loss camp

Many parents send their children to summer weight loss camps. But how good are these camps, and what do they have to offer? Perhaps not all that those concerned about children would like.

"Most camps are costly, stress excessive weight loss and fail to include an intensive family component," says Laurel Mellin, RD, Director of the Center for Adolescent Obesity, San Francisco.

Mellin says the typically severe dietary restrictions at the camps actually stimulate binge eating after camp is over, and it may foster weight gain through biological changes. Also, since the family has not made concomitant changes to support the teenager's new lifestyle, it is not likely to continue and weight regain is likely.

Such camps, Mellin points out, "are most likely to attract families that are desperate about their adolescent's weight and want to have their child fixed. The obese adolescent becomes the victim as parents first delight in initial weight loss, then despair and blame him or her as weight regain predictably occurs."

While some camping programs recognize the vulnerability of young people and employ qualified health professionals, others do not. These often rely on lay staff who focus too much on exercise and rigid and overly restrictive diets. Young people at summer camps may be especially vulnerable to unfortunate weight loss experiences, Mellin suggests.[19]

China seems to have taken the weight loss camp to the extreme. The Associated Press recently told of a 10-day weight loss camp for

60 children, ages 8 to 14, directed by Dr. Yan Chun, chief endocrinologist at Beijing Children's Hospital.

Yan restricted his young campers to an 800 to 1,000 calorie, high protein, low starch, no-sweets diet. He exercised them four to five hours per day, and medicated them with a "new appetite suppressant."

The program "seems to be working," the reporter concluded, because "the children's main topic of conversation was how much fat they'd shed."[20]

Laxatives and diuretics

Taking laxatives or diuretics is a dangerous and ineffective way to lose weight. In the Cleveland study African American girls were the most likely to use laxatives and diuretics — 18 percent had used laxatives and 11 percent diuretics in attempts to lose weight. About half of users took these pills every month or more often.[21] But laxatives and diuretics were more common among Hispanic and white girls in the 1995 Youth Risk Behavior Survey, (11 percent and 8 percent) than black girls (4 percent).

Laxative abuse can cause both acute and chronic lower gastrointestinal complications, including abdominal cramping, bloating, pain, nausea, constipation and diarrhea, say Amy Baker Dennis, PhD, and Randy Sansone, MD, in their "Overview of eating disorders," written for the National Eating Disorders Organization.[22]

Superficially, laxatives cause weight loss through chronic dehydration due to a large volume of watery diarrhea, explain University of Colorado eating disorder specialists Philip Mehler and Kenneth Weiner. Calorie absorption is not really affected. However, nutrients such as protein and calcium may be poorly absorbed.[23]

Mehler and Weiner say that laxative abuse may also cause malabsorption of fat, protein and calcium. Laxatives can result in the loss of electrolytes, including potassium, which is essential for heart function. As potassium level drops, the likelihood of heart arrhythmias increases.

Chronic abuse may cause nerve damage resulting in sluggish bowel function. This happens as the colon becomes thin, dilated and lacking in normal propulsive action, and can become so severe that removal of the colon is needed, to be replaced by a colectomy.

Tolerance develops over time to laxatives and instead of the usual dose of one or two tablets only, abusers often take up to 60 or more tablets daily. Laxatives are probably the most common type of drug abused by bulimic patients, eating disorder specialists say.[24]

Diuretics or "water pills" are used less often by youngsters, but this abuse is extremely dangerous. The big concern here is potassium loss in heart arrhythmia as well as kidney damage. Diuretic abuse can cause rapid and dramatic potassium loss and dehydration.

Using several purging techniques together can intensify the over-all effects on potassium and fluid loss. A physician should be consulted immediately if there are any signs of potassium loss, such as muscle weakness, fatigue and chest pain.

Herbal teas

Herbal weight loss teas can cause fatalities, too, warns the FDA.[25]

Of particular concern were reports to FDA of at least four deaths in women who drank Laci Le Beau Super Dieter's Tea. All died suddenly, and three of the four had cardiac effects. All used the tea at least several times a week.

Similar teas the FDA studied were Trim-Maxx, 24-Hour Diet Tea, and Ultra Slim Tea. Adverse effects reported from these teas ranged from diarrhea, cramps, fainting and permanent loss of bowel function, to death.

The teas often contain large doses of stimulant laxatives such as the herbs senna, cascara, castor oil, buckthorn, aloe and rhubarb root, alone or in combination. These are often used in over-the-counter laxatives — but in smaller, well-controlled dosages.

Since the teas are sold as food supplements, the exact amounts of laxative in each tea are unknown, as are the effects of mixing different laxative herbs. Potency can vary widely with the growing season, amount used in the tea, and length of time the tea is steeped.

Bee pollen, too, has caused fatal allergic reactions. FDA warns that — although promoters claim it is "naturally safe" and "safe for any dieter" — bee pollen holds hazards for anyone with allergies, asthma or hay fever.[26]

Authorities in Australia recently linked royal bee jelly to a severe asthma attack that killed an 11-year-old girl.[27]

Vomiting

In a desperate effort to lose weight, some kids vomit. It's a method that seems to be common among white girls, used by about one in five in the Cleveland study.[28]

Vomiting is a purging behavior that can cause many medical complications including sore throat, heartburn-like pain, esophageal rupture, tooth decay, loss of potassium, dehydration and cardiac arrhythmias.[29]

Irritating the upper gastrointestinal tract irritation may result in sore throats, difficulty in swallowing and indigestion. Forceful vomiting may cause small tears in the mucosa of the gastrointestinal tract with blood in the vomitus. Occasionally, the force of vomiting can break small blood vessels in the eyes, and injury to the esophageal sphincter, allowing stomach contents into the lower esophagus. The esophagus can rupture after ingestion of a large meal and subsequent forceful vomiting. This is a medical emergency with very severe upper abdominal pain, worsened by swallowing and breathing. It has a high death rate if left untreated; surgery is usually needed.

Prolonged vomiting may cause loss of potassium, an electrolyte, essential for muscle and heart functioning. Low levels can trigger cardiac arrhythmias.

Induced vomiting can cause so-called "chipmunk" cheeks, probably due to repeated stimulation of these glands by the acid contents of the stomach. These swollen facial glands usually go down with cessation of vomiting, but in some cases they may be difficult to reduce and can cause a worsening of the person's cosmetic self-image.

Some kids use Ipecac syrup to induce vomiting. Large doses are extremely dangerous and can cause cardiovascular, gastrointestinal and neuromuscular toxicity.[30]

Those who vomit three times a week or more will eventually show erosion of tooth enamel from the frequent presence of acid vomitus in the mouth. This has been reported after only six months, but can take several years. Teeth become sensitive to heat or cold, develop spaces between, lose fillings and generally deteriorate.

Dieting and fasting

Defined in various ways, dieting may refer to restricting foods or fat, or to following a specific plan with a moderate or very low level of calories. The 1995 Youth Risk Behavior survey found over half of white girls, 53 percent, had dieted to lose weight or keep from gaining in the previous 30 days, along with 48 percent of Hispanic and 32 percent of black girls. Among boys these figures were: Hispanic, 23 percent; white, 16 percent; black, 12 percent.

Dieting and fasting can be extremely detrimental to mental and physical growth and development.

"Dieting is not just about eating, it is an entire way of life," warns Janet Polivy, PhD, a University of Toronto professor who has researched the detrimental effects of dieting for over 20 years. "Life has a different meaning for people when they become dieters. Their self-image and self-esteem is all tied up in this."

Polivy says the dangers of dieting include emotional and psychological harm, eating disorders, financial cost and diminished lifestyle. Her research shows dieters respond differently than non-dieters in a range of situations.

Chronic dieters are easily upset, emotional, have mood swings, are more likely to eat when anxious, and have trouble concentrating on the task at hand if there is any kind of distraction. They are compliant and have a need for perfection, are preoccupied with weight and body dissatisfaction, have lost touch with internal signals of hunger and satiety and rely on cognitive cues for eating. They salivate more when faced with attractive food, and have higher levels of digestive hormones and elevated levels of free fatty acids in their blood. They can go longer without food and eat less under "ideal" circumstances than nondieters, but once started, they binge or eat more, then experience guilt.

A chronic dieter focuses on food, eating and weight, both for herself and in her perception of others, has lower self-esteem, is eager to please and complies with what others ask of her.[31]

Ellyn Satter says that dieting causes a child to cross the line to external restriction of food, leaving behind his or her natural weight regulation and normal responses to internal cues of hunger and satiety.

This is a profound change in eating and has serious consequences. The child learns to distrust his or her own responses and relies instead on external factors such as calorie level, patterns of food selection, lists of dos and dont's, and body weight.

But even so, the internal processes will not be ignored, she warns.

"You have to invest more and more time and effort in overcoming them. I am talking about the physical and emotional symptoms of energy deficit: hunger, increased appetite, fatigue, lethargy, irritability and depression. You have to deprive yourself of eating enough and of eating some kinds of food you like. And you become preoccupied with food and with yourself. In some cases, these negative feelings become very strong, perhaps because the person is depriving herself terribly, or because she is particularly sensitive to the feelings of deprivation, or because she doesn't lose weight very easily and she just keeps trying harder and harder. When this happens, she has a choice: she can either decide the juice isn't worth the squeeze and go back to eating normally (or at least dieting less harshly), or she can intensify her efforts."[32]

"Although weight/shape concerns and dieting behavior are common in elementary school children . . . they are not harmless," point out Linda Smolak and Michael Levine, eating disorder specialists at Kenyon College in Gambier, Ohio.

"In the short run, caloric-restrictive diets generate irritability, distractibility, food preoccupation and fatigue. The longterm effects are more worrisome. Dieting children may be at special risk for developing severe eating disorders . . . Caloric restriction during childhood and adolescence can lead to stunted growth, menstrual dysfunction and decreased bone density."[33]

One chronic dieter, who did not have an eating disorder, says dieting makes her less of a human being. "What I resent about dieting is that it makes one so terribly self-centered, so much aware of oneself and one's body, so preoccupied with things that apply to oneself only, that there is scarcely any energy left to be really spontaneous, relaxed and outgoing. It starts with thinking about what to eat and what not to eat, and gradually goes over to other fields, and it is this aspect that makes me resent dieting; it makes me less of a human being."[34]

"Dieting shrinks a woman's world, not her body," adds Merryl Bear, Co-ordinator of the National Eating Disorder Information Centre in Toronto.[35]

Dieting is abnormal

The problem with dieting is that we are not able to integrate diet behavior into our normal lifestyle because it is abnormal, says Mary Evans Young, the founder of No Diet Day, and author of *Diet Breaking.*

"Dieting is based on deprivation, sacrifice and guilt, which are difficult to sustain. We lose touch with our natural hunger signals in responding to external cues which don't address underlying issues." [36]

Diets wreck lives, undermine health, sap confidence self-esteem and energy. Dieting affects nearly all girls and women, diverting them from facing their real issues, prevent them from fulfilling their potential, and cause obsession with food, body and weight.[37]

The diet industry has the perfect product, Evans Young observes. "It promises so much, and when it doesn't deliver the consumer blames herself and then goes on to the next diet."

Yet dieting can make girls feel that they are doing the right thing. They feel good just for having made the decision to go on a diet. Pursuing thinness is widely perceived to be the same as pursuing good health.

"That feeling of self-sacrifice can hook us into wonderful feelings of purity and goodness," notes Evans Young. "The diet becomes a kind of fanatical religion, requiring you to abide by a set of stringent rules or pay the penance of guilt. It's a guilt that starts by slowly nibbling and then steadily gnaws away at your body, spirit and confidence. Give yourself a break. You deserve much, much more."[38]

Semi-starvation diets

Diets of less than 900 calories offer special appeal because dieters initially lose appetite and weight drops off rapidly for a time. But they carry serious health risks, even when under medical supervision. The risks escalate when children and teens engage in do-it-yourself types of fasting, fad diets and liquid diets.

One of the highest risks for sudden death syndrome in weight loss is during very low calorie diets, warn researchers at the National Institutes of Health Obesity Research Center in New York. However, there can be fatal cardiac arrhythmias, apparently related to the shrinking size of heart muscle that parallels the large, rapid weight losses of a very low calorie diet.

Rapid weight loss increases also gallstone risk. Children rarely develop gallstones, but a 13-year-old girl had to have her gallbladder removed after losing weight through a diet prescribed by the Doctors Quick Weight Loss Center. Her mother, Loretta Pameijer, testified at the 1990 congressional subcommittee hearings on the weight loss industry. The girl was given a cursory physical plus a test for food allergies before beginning the program. Then she was given a food chart that supposedly reflected the allergy test results and listed foods the girl could and couldn't eat.

Although her daughter followed the diet faithfully, there were times when she would stop losing weight, Pameijer said. "The counselors would put her on a parsley break. It had almost nothing in it but meat and a half a cup of parsley a day."

The girl's physician said she had "the worst gallbladder attack" he had ever seen in anyone so young.

"We're angry because it never occurred to us to be suspicious of a doctors' clinic," Pameijer said.

The New York investigation also turned up numerous injuries, including the case of a 15-year-old Long Island girl who had to have her gallbladder removed after losing 72 pounds in six months.

University of Alabama nutrition researchers find new gallstones form in 10 to 26 percent of persons on very low calorie diets and may occur within four weeks.[39]

Risks of dieting and weight loss

Mental and emotional risks

- Apathy
- Depression, anxiety
- Irritability, intolerance, moodiness
- Decrease in mental alertness, comprehension, and concentration
- Thoughts focused on eating, weight and hunger
- Self-absorbed, self-focused, decrease in wider interests
- Preoccupation with own body, judgmental of size of others
- Lowered self-esteem, feels self-worth depends on being thin

Physical risks

- Weakness, fainting, fatigue
- Cold intolerance
- Gallstones
- Gouty arthritis
- Cardiac disorders
- Elevated cholesterol
- Anemia
- Headache
- Elevated uric acid levels
- Loss of lean tissue
- Nausea
- Diarrhea, constipation
- Edema
- Hair loss and thinning hair
- Hypotension
- Abdominal pain
- Muscle cramps
- Aching muscles
- Both slowed and increased heart rate
- Heart abnormalities, arrhythmias
- Sudden death

HEALTH RISKS OF WEIGHT LOSS, 1995

Treatment for large children

Large children and teens may be put on semi-starvation very low calorie diets of under 800 calories, treated with appetite suppressant drugs, or subjected to gastric surgery. The goals are to achieve longterm weight loss without doing physical or emotional harm to the child. But there is little evidence of these goals being achieved.

Treatment programs for large children and adolescents traditionally have emphasized food restraint and control. Such a focus dwells on negative behavior rather than positive, even though most have added an exercise component in the past decade.

Some of these treatments are conservative, recommending a gradual weight loss of approximately a pound a week or so. Others are severe and cause large, rapid, short-term weight loss.

Although there is much less support for rigid diets today, many authorities still recommend them. Regretfully, the prestigious 1995 book, *Weighing the Options*, by the Food and Nutrition Board of the Institute of Medicine, recommends dieting as the way to help large children.

"Dieting remains the cornerstone of therapy for the obese child since caloric restriction produces far greater energy deficits than exercise alone," advises Beatrice Kanders, EdD, RD, in a section on pediatric obesity.

She suggests use of either the low calorie diet or the more restrictive very low calorie diet for children and adolescents.[1] She recommends a liquid diet of 600 to 800 calories, with the addition of two to four cups of low-starch vegetables to make up part of the calories, which she calls a protein-sparing modified fast. The addition of food explains the diet being called a "protein-sparing modified fast," a somewhat outdated term currently being revived. (Now disproved, it was once claimed that this kind of very low calorie diet would cause the loss of fat only, and that "protein" or muscle would be spared.)

Weighing the Options recommends this diet be limited to high-risk cases, the "more serious cases of childhood and adolescent obesity, for which rapid weight reduction is essential.

"In children, the protein-sparing modified fast has been used on children as young as 6 years of age and by children whose body weight ranges from 120 percent to greater than 200 percent of ideal body weight . . . In England, (it) is not recommended for use by children under the age of 13." An average weight loss of about 22 pounds in 10 weeks may be expected, it notes.

Unfortunately, of course, that weight is almost invariably regained quickly. And it is not explained why a large, rapid weight loss, with its potentially severe consequences, followed by rapid regain, can be essential or healthy for "the more serious cases."

Smoking to lose weight

Nicotine is probably the most successful dieting drug of all time, the most common and one of the most dangerous. And smoking among young people, especially girls and women, is rising significantly. If current trends continue, smoking rates for men and women will soon be the same, if not higher for women.[40]

White high school girls are already smoking at rates as high as boys. The reason: to control their weight.

One in three high school students smoke, according to the 1995 Youth Risk Behavior survey. Smoking rates are highest for white students at 38 percent, compared with 34 percent for Hispanic and 19 percent for black students. White girls have the highest rates of all at 40 percent, compared with only 12 percent for black girls. Current use is defined as having smoked at least one cigarette in the past month.

Smoking has its own powerful industry promoting nicotine to children and teenagers as a method of weight control. Women, especially, are a target.

The jump in smoking for young women began during his tenure in the late 1970s, "to the point where for almost two decades teenage girls have been puffing away at rates exceeding or equal to those of teenage boys," admits Joseph Califano, Jr., former secretary of Health, Education and Welfare. He says he regrets that he did not deal with the fear of weight gain early in the fight against smoking to help prevent this.

Targeting women in cigarette advertising began in the late 1960s, he said, and in the next 20 years death rates from lung cancer increased 500 percent for female smokers.

Today, references to slimness appear in nearly all smoking advertisements in magazines aimed at a female audience.[41]

With teenage girls leading the way, 3,000 American adolescents
become regular smokers every day.

"Virtually all will be sicker than the rest of the population, most
will never quit, and more than a third face early death as a consequence of their addiction," says Califano.

He says the nation's obsession with thinness is a great boon to
tobacco companies — they play shrewdly on the fear of weight gain.

"That's what makes Virginia Slims and Capri Superslims —
with their names, slim cigarette outlines, and extremely thin models
— so attractive to teenage girls."

Smoking is also beginning at younger and younger ages, according to the Healthy People 2000 report by the U.S. Public Health
Service. Nearly all new smokers now begin during adolescence. Of

---

What's wrong with dieting?

- Dieting doesn't work, weight is quickly regained

- Dieting is dangerous, causes deaths and injury

- Dieting disrupts normal eating habits

- Dieting can initiate eating disorders

- Dieting stunts children's growth and development

- Dieting diminishes women, diverts dreams and ambition

- Dieting saps strength and energy

- Dieting is expensive, but without value

- Dieting causes obsessive food preoccupation

- Dieting increases prejudice against large persons

high school students who have ever smoked, about one-quarter smoked their first cigarette by grade 6, one-half by grade 8, and three-fourths by grade 9. Most adult smokers started to smoke regularly before age 20.[42]

Those who start smoking early have more difficulty quitting, are more likely to become heavy smokers, and are more likely to develop a smoking-related disease, says this report.

The tobacco industry denies that it targets children and adolescents. But cigarette advertising is heavy in many magazines with large adolescent readerships and uses the kind of image-based ads which are most effective with young people. This kind of imagery is tested to have its greatest impact on children and lower socioeconomic groups.

Tobacco companies also sponsor sporting events, rock concerts, and other competitions which attract young people and get wide television coverage. Television brings these events into the nation's living rooms, along with tobacco company names and logos, helping to deliver the youth market to the sponsors. Violation of codes that prohibit sale of cigarettes to minors or giving free cigarette samples to youth is widespread.

Tobacco is responsible for more than one of every six deaths in the U.S., according to the Healthy People 2000 report. It is the most important single preventable cause of death and disease in this country. Cigarette smoking directly accounts for about 390,000 deaths yearly including 21 percent of all coronary heart disease deaths, 87 percent of lung cancer deaths, and 30 percent of all cancer deaths.

Smoking during pregnancy accounts for 20 to 30 percent of low birth weight babies, up to 14 percent of preterm deliveries, and about 10 percent of all infant deaths.

Girls and women are not as likely to quit smoking as are males.

Numerous studies confirm the popular belief that smoking does help to keep weight down, and upon quitting smoking, most people gain some weight.[43] This effect is well-known to teenagers.

Smokers who quit in the past 10 years gained an average of 11 pounds for women and 10 pounds for men above the weight gain of those who continued smoking, in the NHANES III studies by the health department. But their weight did not differ from that of persons who had never smoked. This is consistent with other studies that show people who quit smoking "catch up" in weight with their peers who did not begin smoking.[44]

Thus, nicotine acts much like the new prescription appetite suppressant pills. Such drugs help the patient lose a certain number of pounds, which are kept off as long as the drug is being taken and regained when the drug is withdrawn.

The Healthy People 2000 goal is to reduce smoking by children and youth so that no more than 15 percent have become regular cigarette smokers by age 20. With the public health pressure on children to lose weight, it is doubtful they will respond to this goal.

CHAPTER 9

New health promoting
model needed

■

As these problems claim more and more children, it's time for a new approach. What we've been doing is not working well. More children eat abnormally. More children live with eating disorders. More struggle with overweight. More are contemplating suicide. More fail to thrive because of the social shame they endure for being fat.

While these problems may be more acute for American children, they are shared in many other countries throughout the world.

It's time to throw out the old model. These aren't separate issues, they're all part of the same problem and they're all influenced by our unnatural obsession with thinness. In the new paradigm, we deal with these issues in healthy ways. The goal is to encourage the healthy growth and development of the whole child — his or her emotional, mental, physical, intellectual, spiritual and social development — and it includes every child of every size.

We need to help young people build self-esteem, learn assertiveness and healthy coping skills. We want them to develop their unique potential as lovable, capable, valuable individuals, and take pride in themselves and their bodies at any size, without being stigmatized.

We must change the focus from dieting to being healthy at the weight we are. There's much evidence that keeping a stable weight through adult life is healthier than losing and gaining weight, even for large persons.

The unifying approach

So what do we do?

We need a shared vision and consistent messages that communicate this vision.

The unifying approach is a new, health promoting way of preventing and dealing with weight and eating problems. As shown here *(fig. 1)*, this approach is based on the principles of good health for every person of every size. Families, community leaders, educators, health care providers and health policy are united in the goal of promoting good health that does no harm, recognizing the interrelatedness of the four major problems. In this way, we will solve problems rather than create new ones. A united effort can also act on the culture in positive ways, and respond effectively to its negative pressures.

The underlying unity in this approach is that what is healthy for the largest child in school is also healthy for the thinnest. It's a way that does no harm to either child.

When we focus on one or two problems to the detriment of others, healthy living is sacrificed. When the focus is on reducing overweight alone, there is high probability of intensifying the problems of dysfunctional eating, dangerous weight loss methods, eating disorders, and the stigmatization of larger kids. When the focus is solely on eating disorder, the dangers of promoting weight loss are known, but not the problems of excessive weight gain. When self-esteem is ignored, when the power of society is brushed off, then we see more kids contemplating suicide.

Appallingly the public is even being told that self-acceptance is not acceptable if one is large, as in the influential new report *Weighing the Options*, which warns, "It is inappropriate to argue that obese individuals should simply accept their body weight and not try to reduce."

This sets one policy against another, and it violates the principle to do no harm. Health professionals, educators and parents need to look carefully at all the problems, aware of the harm that can and is being done to vulnerable children and teens, and find positive ways of working together to build strengths in these areas. Those who set national health policy, in particular need to take a broader look at weight and eating problems.

Changing national policy would make a difference, since it sets much of the agenda for what happens throughout the country. It also profoundly influences the media's focus in health issues.

By taking the unified approach, we recognize that today's problems include the high prevalence of obesity, the risks of obesity, and the failure of weight loss treatment. They include eating disorders and their effects, pressures to be extremely thin, the high rates and impact of disturbed eating on young people, the health risks of weight

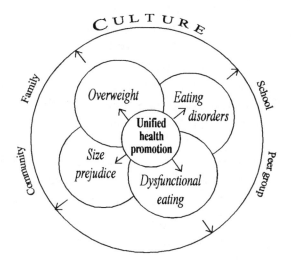

Figure 1

Health promotion approach

A unified approach focuses on good health for all children, does no harm, recognizes the interrelatedness of eating and weight problems, and strengthens the positive aspects of culture, family, friends.[1]

Afraid to Eat 1997

loss and dieting, size prejudice and the stigmatization of large persons, and the women's issues which severely affect body image for many young girls.

The unified health promotion approach seeks not only to decrease the prevalence of these problems, but to encourage healthy living at any weight and to shape public policy to these ends. It also seeks to keep a balanced perspective which weighs the many related issues across the weight spectrum and the need to find healthful solutions for all.

Community coalitions

Most important, we can bring about positive change by uniting health policy and institutions with family, school and community, so that all work together in nurturing our children.

The community approach provides families with a supportive, caring network of friends in raising their children. It creates the kind of informal associations that previous generations of parents depended on for support and guidance. The need for an integrated school and community approach is being rediscovered as an effective way to promote good health for young people.

Communities across the country are discovering new energy in working toward a positive vision for young people through a Minneapolis-based program called "Healthy communities, healthy youth" by Search Institute.[1]

This is an initiative that motivates communities to make better use of existing organizations and institutions. Instead of focusing in a negative way on problems such as violence or drugs, then getting federal funding and hiring experts to fix them — which tends to cause more alienation and isolation in the community — it calls for a shift to positive action.

The goal is to create a way of life in communities where all young people are valued and valuable, problems are more manageable, and an attitude of vision, hope and celebration pervades community life.

This approach shifts attention from problems to working toward a common vision of what is needed to promote the healthy development of young people. The program involves churches, civic and school organizations, businesses and individuals. It thrives from the inspiration, passion and gifts of individuals and groups doing what they can to build assets in young people. All residents see themselves as guardians of the community's young people.

It's a positive action to reverse the crumbling infrastructure of neighborhoods all across the country.

The asset-building Search approach can help parents be consistent in their choices with other community efforts, knowing their decisions can have a tremendously positive impact in shaping their children's lives. They are reinforced in teaching the values and priorities they wish to pass on to their children. Parents feel supported.

"The community is filled with consistent messages," says Peter Benson, president of Search Institute. "If you spend time in an asset-building community, you quickly sense harmony in the messages that young people hear . . . People consistently hear that young people are a priority in the community."

The local media repeatedly communicate the vision in these communities, support local mobilization efforts, and provide forums for sharing innovative actions.

A new paradigm

This new paradigm shifts the emphasis away from weight loss, and toward self-trust, empowerment, self-acceptance, and preventing problems. It encourages children to eat, move and grow in normal ways, working with their natural regulatory abilities. It promotes natural, wholesome eating patterns, healthy food relationships and regular physical activities, to set the stage in childhood for healthy lifestyles to enable them to maintain a natural and stable weight through life.

This new paradigm or new perspective is being called the health promotion approach. It grows out of the nondiet movement, a movement led by nutritionists, health professionals and consumers that advocates normal eating and rejects the promotion of dysfunctional eating that's inherent in dieting and most weight loss programs. It challenges traditional thinking that everyone should be thin, and that large people should be always trying to lose weight, and instead encourages them to maintain a healthy, active lifestyle, feel good about themselves, and keep a stable weight.

Ellyn Satter, MS, RD, a registered dietitian, family therapist and well-known authority on feeding infants and children, is a national leader in this new approach. She explains, "The emerging paradigm is a trust paradigm, based on observations that children have tendencies for a particular body build, including the food regulation processes and inclinations for movement that support those tendencies. The task for the growing child is not to remain slim, but to maintain energy balance in response to variations in caloric density of the diet, activity level and growth."

The new thinking understands the severity of the problem for youth, especially adolescent girls, many of whom have arrested their physical and intellectual development while trying to reshape their bodies to what they believe is most socially acceptable.

Growing up large is acceptable

Many — perhaps most — nutritionists, including dietitians, now accept the new paradigm. They were among the first professionals to revise their traditional role in weight loss treatment.

At the front of this movement is Satter who has untiringly presented her innovative ideas to nutrition leaders for over 10 years. She published *How to Get Your Kid to Eat...But Not Too Much*, in 1987, expanding on the ideas in her ground-breaking 1983 book, *Child of Mine: Feeding with Love and Good Sense*.

The new thinking took root and is now reflected in American Dietetic Association position papers, and policy decisions of the Society for Nutrition Education, which recently formed a special member section on Weight Realities.

Leaders in the new movement are committed to helping people understand that the body cannot be shaped at will. That individual differences in body shapes and sizes are natural and desirable. That weight which evolves naturally from healthy lifestyle needs to be accepted.

And yes, these leaders are willing to accept what has long been unacceptable: that obese youngsters may not achieve permanent weight loss or grow up to be thin. The new guidelines and programs recognize this and deal with it in a straightforward manner.

"There is no reason your child cannot lead a happy, productive, full life at whatever size she turns out to be," explains Joanne Ikeda, MA, RD, a California nutrition education specialist with the Cooperative Extension Service, University of California, Berkeley, and leader in the size acceptance movement.[2]

Canada's *Vitality* program puts it this way: "To overcome the influence of a media-dominated culture that judges women on how they look, we must encourage women to accept a wide range of healthy body weights and shapes, to love their bodies as they are, to value slimness only as it relates to overall health, to refrain from dieting and to reject societal pressures to conform to an unrealistic body size. In doing so, women will improve their self-images and be more realistic in their assessment of body image.

"One of the results of living in a thinness culture is the belief that health is improved with weight loss and achieving a low body weight. This basic assumption has been challenged and the negative effects of dieting and weight cycling are now being examined closely.

Health promotion paradigm

Preventing weight and eating problems through:
- trust, empowerment
- normal eating balanced by active living
- encouraging stable weights
- self-acceptance
- appreciation of diversity, accepting a wider range of shapes and sizes

Canadian *Vitality* message:
  "Eat well, be active and feel good about yourself."

The shift to *Vitality* from a weight centered approach

Weight centered approach	VITALITY

DIETING

- Restrictive eating
- Counting calories, prescriptive diets
- Weight cycling (yo-yo diets)
- Eating disorders

HEALTHY EATING

- Take pleasure in eating a variety of foods
- Enjoy lower-fat, complex-carbo-hydrate foods more often
- Meet the body's energy and nutrient needs through a lifetime of healthy, enjoyable eating
- Take control of how you eat by listening to your hunger cues

EXERCISE

- No pain, no gain
- Prescriptions such as three times a week in your target heart-rate zone
- Burn calories
- High attrition rates for vigorous exercise programs

ACTIVE LIVING

- Value and practice activities that are moderate and fun
- Be active your way, every day
- Participate for the joy of feeling your body move• Enjoy physical activities as part of your daily lifestyle

DISSATISFACTION WITH SELF

- Unrealistic goals for body size and shape
- Obsession and preoccupation with weight
- Fat phobia and discrimination against overweight people
- Striving to be a perfect "10" and to maintain an impossible "ideal" (thin or muscular) body size
- Accepting the fashion, diet and tobacco industries' emphasis on slimness

POSITIVE SELF/BODY IMAGE

- Accept and recognize that healthy bodies come in a range of weights, shapes/sizes
- Appreciate your strengths and abilities
- Be tolerant of a wide range of body sizes and shapes
- Relax and enjoy the unique characteristics you have to offer
- Be critical of messages that focus on unrealistic thinness (in women) and muscularity (in men) as symbols of success and happiness

The VITALITY approach calls for a shift from negative to positive thinking about how to achieve and maintain healthy weights.[2]

"While a reduction in weight will improve the health of some overweight people, a fixation on weight reduction and ideal body shape can lead to yo-yo dieting, weight cycling, restrictive eating, obsessive exercising and negative perceptions of body image. Furthermore, pursuit of a rigid standard for size and shape inevitably fails for most people over the long term."

Programs based on the new paradigm offer a fresh approach that is flexible, open, accepting, individualized and family-centered. But above all, they focus on the whole child, and on every child as a valued human being. They consider each as an individual with all his or her complexities and contradictions.

Such programs appreciate the local culture and family traditions and values. Parents are assured that they can trust their family traditions, that these are valuable to pass down through the generations, shaped and expressed in different ways as they may be, yet honoring the past. They are encouraged to trust their judgment, to feel confident that they and their children can make good decisions. Parents who are confused and shaken by confusing health messages, need to learn to trust themselves again.

The message is "trust yourself." Trust and empower the child. Support the child in solving his or her own problems, even when that child marches to a different drummer.

Canada and Vitality

Canadian educators and health professionals have succeeded in developing a national policy, a national way of thinking that focuses on health instead of weight. I began talking with leaders in the Canadian movement in the late 1980s. They discovered me first as readers of *Healthy Weight Journal*, and started sending their innovative ideas my way.

Heather Nielsen, Chief of Nutrition Programs at Health Canada in Ottawa, first sent me papers from major meetings that discussed — right along with the problems of obesity — eating disorders, preoccupation with weight and negative body image (a bridging taboo frowned on in Washington). It was a new way to advance knowledge and understanding I hadn't seen before.

Then these bold Canadians tore apart the sacrosanct height-weight tables and worked out some broad ranges. Finally, they more or less shelved the healthy weight ranges, too, and gave us an eloquent concept: *Vitality*.

After years of meetings and lengthy discussions by dozens of eminent experts, Vitality is simplicity itself. It tells Canadians — and people all over the world — to enjoy eating well, being active and feeling good about yourself.

Vitality is an integrated approach to healthy living that shifts the focus away from rigid ideals, dieting and prescriptive exercise toward an acceptance of a variety of body sizes and shapes and an emphasis on healthy eating, active living and positive self and body image.

The message is to be healthy at the weight you are, get on with life, and stop obsessing about your weight. It's a message of preventing problems before they happen.

Vitality is also the basis for new treatment programs with its three-pronged approach of eating well, living actively and feeling good. School programs emphasize nondieting, eating normally, improving self-esteem and dealing with size discrimination.[3]

Canada included women eating disorder specialists who embrace the new paradigm as an important part of the decision-making team. However, in the U.S., such specialists, are seldom included in health policy planning.

I've been so enthusiastic about Vitality, that at one point Heather Nielsen and I went to Washington, D.C, where I was pleased and honored be able to set up a presentation for a nutrition group and invited public health officials. The nutritionists loved it, but it had no discernible effect on health policy. Maybe we planted seeds. But it seemed to me, rather, that it strengthened resistance to change within a closed circle.

Political changes needed

The United States has to change its health policy in this arena. Eating disorders must be added to the nation's health agenda for Healthy People 2000 revisions. The total picture, which includes obesity, eating disorders, dysfunctional eating, discrimination against large persons, must be considered in attempting to deal with weight and eating problems. Only when all the issues are allowed on the table, can a comprehensive policy be developed which makes sense and which health professionals will support.

Considering the four problems together as interrelated problems with an awareness of how they affect each other, being wary of the harm so easily done to vulnerable youth, is the way to bring us to the health promoting solutions needed. The new approach keeps this in perspective. It challenges the detrimental effects of traditional thinking and health policies aimed at size alone, not the effect on the whole person. All these factors are in the mix when we consider the complex areas of weight and eating, and what they mean in our culture.

As we search for answers, it is well to remember that weight, eating, and even health are only a small part of what makes life worthwhile. We need to keep a balanced perspective. Wellness and wholeness are not about attaining perfect health, or even longevity, but improving the quality of life and living well.

What we need is for our leaders — health providers, educators, community leaders, parents — to embrace and teach the concept of wellness and wholeness, which is a healing and nourishing of the mind, body and spirit.

New leaders

The good news is this new way of dealing with weight problems is already moving ahead. We are in the midst of a new movement that will not be stopped. Diets that don't work, pressures to be thin, and crises in disturbed eating — these are all reasons why women are responding with excitement to what has been called the nondiet movement.

It now embodies much more than nondiet — it's a health promoting approach that replaces the weight loss approach. Health, not reaching a so-called ideal weight, is the focus.

"It means listening to your body," writes Linda Omichinski, author of *You Count, Calories Don't*. "It means discovering individual patterns for food and activity levels that keep you energized. It means finding the strength to accept yourself just as you are and get on with life."

Women are in the forefront of this new movement. And this makes a great deal of sense. Women know the issues. They are well aware of how disproportionately young girls suffer from eating disorders, dysfunctional eating, and the stigma of overweight. They have struggled with their own weight and body issues, and understand the problems well. Mostly they are professionals, in fields related to nutrition, eating disorders, and size acceptance. They are educators, extension agents, authors, health providers, mothers. They are also joined by many supportive men.

Many of them live in Canada, where new, healthier attitudes are encouraged by national policy. It is initiated by Health Canada, and has brought about tremendous changes in schools, community and the health care.

It's been my privilege to network with many of these new leaders for a number of years. I've been inspired by their new, healthier treatment programs and approaches to problems, and pleased that they've been inspired by my writing. It's also been a delight and something of a surprise to have become a rallying point for size acceptance groups from all over the world.

There is even a feminist perspective to all this, although these women would not call themselves "feminists" (perhaps some will move into positions vacated by leaders in the feminist movement, who, it has been said, are too busy dieting). They point out that dieting and semi-starvation keep women preoccupied and passive, off career ambitions, and that women are dehumanized by their portrayal in the media, advertising and the fashion industry.

We must change our culture. We have to challenge, speak out, sometimes boycott that which exceeds the bounds of being friendly to our society. Working together, we can do this. We can shift the focus away from restrictive ideals, dieting, and prejudice, toward healthier goals. We are in the process of defining healthy weight, in ways it has not been defined before. We can rally women of all sizes and all walks of life to appreciate their own diversity — whether in the thinnest five percent or the largest.

Together we can do this hard and vital thing that needs doing, women everywhere, with the help of the wonderful male allies who are in this struggle along with their wives, daughters, mothers.

The new health promotion movement is growing and it is being embraced by many federal researchers and scientists, parents, teachers and the general public. Working together and supported by a unifying health policy, our families, schools, communities and health care providers can bring about the healthy change that is needed.

CHAPTER 10

In the family

■

Families are crucial to defusing this public health crisis in which children are afraid to eat.

Parents can help their children restore normal eating, and the sooner, the better. The longer they struggle with eating and weight issues, the more dysfunctional these can become. And the more likely that the issues will deteriorate into more severe problems. If an eating disorder is suspected it's important to have the problem evaluated by a competent therapist and if needed, to get the child into therapy without delay.

Yet it is easy to add to the anxiety, fear and pressure these kids are already feeling. Parents need to maintain a low key approach, avoid increasing the tensions, and focus on supporting the child with love and acceptance. Families with healthy attitudes and behavior are at the heart of promoting healthy growth and development for their children.

Mothers and fathers who are obsessed or worried over their own weight, continually dieting, restricting fat or calories, and often talking about these concerns, can set up their children for eating problems at very young ages. A parent's overconcern about a child's weight further adds to the tension, fear and confusion that child is feeling.

Families need to be safe places where children are loved and accepted unconditionally, as beautiful and capable individuals. But parents often don't know how to deal with a child who is struggling with dysfunctional eating, an eating disorder, overweight or size prejudice.

Children are crying out for help and support from their families. I receive heartbreaking letters from teenagers who are struggling to cope with weight and eating pressures in their lives. Many of them write about communicating: I can't talk to my parents; they're too busy; they won't listen; they don't understand; they want to run my life; they say it's nothing, to forget it.

What can I tell them? I'm a parent and I've made mistakes. I'm not a therapist.

But I tell them you are lovable, beautiful and capable just as you are. I hope you'll come to accept yourself, and believe in yourself. Learning acceptance will help release the tension that you say is taking over your life and threatening to tear apart your family.

And please stop those thoughts of suicide. You said you didn't want to hurt your parents, but this is a permanent way to hurt them badly for the rest of their lives. You can interrupt your negative thoughts and replace them with pleasant images if you'll work on it. I hope you will.

Find someone to talk to — your parents, your therapist, a school counsellor, a pastor or priest. Talking about how you feel will help.

It's sad that you, and kids like you, are being made to feel you have to meet some "perfect" standards to be loved and accepted. Our country needs to appreciate diversity again and not focus so much on physical appearance.

You are okay just as you are. Tall is nice, short is nice — so is large or small, or being attractive or not so attractive. This is the way life is. It's us, all of us, the human race in all its wonderful diversity.

I know this tolerance isn't being shown right now, especially in the media, and I'm sorry. But I have faith it will change. You and I, your mom and dad, our friends, working together, we can make changes in what our culture seems to be expecting of kids.

Restore normal eating

An emphasis on sound, healthy lifestyles is the best known prevention for weight and eating problems, overweight and underweight as well as the range of eating disorders.

As in the Canadian Vitality healthy weight programs, the family focus should be on eating well, living actively and feeling good about yourself and others.

"Vitality is a shift in thinking about what healthy living really is. It's a lifestyle for everyone. It's throwing a Frisbee with the kids, having friends over for a potluck dinner, curling up and enjoying a good book. It's about healthy eating and active living. It's gardening and cycling, laughing and relaxing. It's good for you — body and soul."

Mothers, fathers and children who feel good about themselves and each other make healthy choices easy — not just for a short period of time but for a lifetime.

Restoration of normal eating is a priority for all youth who have restricted their eating out of fear of fat, as well as for those who habitually overeat. This begins with restoring normal eating patterns where they are erratic, not only for the child, but for all others in the family.

Unfortunately, today many parents are so confused and fearful of their own eating, weight and health, that their fears are multiplied in their children.

Mothers and fathers need to examine their own attitudes and behaviors, and consider whether they may be contributing to their children's eating and weight problems. Parents with dysfunctional eating patterns need to make healthy changes in their own and family eating practices. In doing this, it is helpful to avoid much discussion or thinking about weight and diet.

Family communication

It's important that families talk to each other, especially about feelings, in order to get them out in the open and deal with them in healthy ways. Some parents are afraid or don't know how to express their own feelings. They're afraid they'll be unable to help or know the right answers, so they don't allow their children to express their feelings.

Communication builds relationships. It lets moms and dads know what their kids are doing and thinking. It helps kids understand who their parents are. It lays a foundation for positive family life.

Some mothers and fathers need to practice asking, "How do you feel about that?" and then listen, and keep asking and listening, without offering any solutions at all. Trying to solve problems that should be "owned" by the child is controlling and destructive behavior for parents. Instead, parents need to be able to listen in a caring way, and trust the child.

Young people need to feel they can talk about their problems and freely express their feelings without having them taken over and "solved" by their parents. This is especially important for teenagers, who soon stop sharing when this happens. But the foundation for free and open expression is laid in childhood.

Sometimes the problems seem small to a parent — a torn favorite shirt; a friend's snub; missing out on an event. Talking it out can help children keep it small and let it go. It can help them diffuse anger and deal with it in constructive ways. Or it may uncover other, larger problems that need attention.

Sometimes the problem looms so large for the whole family that it is believed too terrible to talk about: mom or dad's alcoholism; gambling; marital discord; an unfortunate incident; physical, sexual or mental abuse.

Children need to know that it is possible to talk about these things. That it's not a good situation, but mom has feelings she can talk about, so does dad, and so does each of the children. When nothing is ever said, the terrible problem grows even worse.

In the case of sexual molestation, children need to know they do not have to put up with this — but too often this is not clear to them. Giving them the words to use and practicing it loud and clear can help: "Don't do that, I don't like it." (This is not to suggest this is the child's problem, it isn't; but it can happen and being prepared can help. Parents and the community are responsible for protecting children from physical, mental and sexual abuse.)

Trying to pretend everything is perfect and conveying the idea that, above all, the family must look perfect in the eyes of neighbors, establishes an impossible standard. This causes enormous stress and sets children up for many kinds of emotional problems.

Often these are expressed in eating disturbances and disorders. Talking about it and expressing feelings diffuses the stress and helps people cope in healthier ways.

Parents who are "too busy" to listen and disengaged parents may need to do some soul-searching about what is really important in their lives. Finding the time and energy to listen at the time it is most needed may be difficult, but it is extremely important in children's lives.

On the other hand, some parents are too controlling, too involved; they need to back off and empower their children by trusting them to make their own good decisions.

It's all part of parenting, giving our children roots and wings.

Caring neighbors

One of the greatest needs of young people is ongoing relationships with caring, principled people. Adults who offer guidance and encouragement, who care about and trust them. They need to have support across the generations, to hear consistent messages about boundaries and values. They need neighbors, relatives, older and younger adults from their schools, churches and communities who call them by name and are their friends.

Many children and teens are missing this support network today. In a survey in Minneapolis, only 29 percent of youth reported experiencing caring neighbors. Many adults have pulled back from offering their support because they feel overwhelmed by today's youth problems that dominate the headlines. Neighbors don't get involved in the lives of children on their block. Often they don't even know their names. They defer to professionals.

The Search program of "Healthy communities, healthy youth" turns this around by urging people to take individual action on their own. Adults are encouraged to do simple things: look at and speak to every child or teen they see; talk to youngsters about their interests; send a birthday or congratulatory card; invite a young person to go along to a ballgame; have an open-door policy so neighbor kids feel welcome to come in for refreshments, conversation, or just hang out. Senior citizens wait for school buses with children, making sure they're safely off to school, while building relationships with children they didn't know before.

Everyone gets involved. Girls on the high school basketball team read to younger children at the library on Saturdays.

It takes effort and time and a commitment to break through barriers. But the rewards of rebuilding the sense of community in our neighborhoods will last for generations.

Youth roles

Search focuses on 40 assets, or building blocks, to help promote the healthy development of children. Surveys show that the more assets young people experience, the more they engage in positive behaviors, such as volunteering and succeeding in school. The fewer they have, the more likely they are to engage in risk-taking behaviors, such as violence, sexual activity, and alcohol and drug use. Each asset is important, and together the benefits are additive.

The goal of a caring community is to increase the number of assets children have, such as:

- Support from three or more non-parent adults.
- Caring neighbors.
- Active, involved parents.
- An attachment to school.
- Desire to help other people.
- Commitment to serve in the community.
- Training in music and the arts.
- Religious participation.
- Skills to resolve conflict non-violently.
- Optimism about his/her personal future.

Children, their families and their neighbors all know these criteria and strive to increase the assets for young people.

This is the kind of action that can bring about healthier families, schools and communities and a child-nurturing, supportive culture for our youth.[1]

Parents need to be aware of the importance of this network of caring adults who help to nurture and support their children. Building and nourishing these relationships is a vital task of parenting. It's especially important now when kids are so heavily influenced by pop culture and the entertainment industries.

The dieting child

How can parents help when a teenager is determined to lose weight? Sometimes all moms and dads can do is go along, help as they can, and ease the stress.

Decisions on what and how much to eat belong to the child; this cannot be infringed.

As a parent of wrestlers, I understand this all too well. Wrestling is a great sport, and I enjoy it. But losing too much weight is a major problem that needs fixing. Our two sons were champion wrestlers in the lower weights and they believed to be champions they had to lose a lot of weight.

With our oldest son Rick, I did everything wrong. His single-minded purpose was so devastating, his level of nutrition so low, and his eating so chaotic, that I felt helpless. I was a nutrition teacher, but I didn't know what to do.

Rick kept eating nonstop candy bars and hot dogs at the gym after a match, and the next day big meals with lots of cookies and snacks, then back to almost nothing the two or three days before the next match. The rest of our family ate as usual. We'd try to coax him to meals, but mostly we tiptoed around and tried not to notice. He'd be kind of irritable after a hard workout, and we learned to leave him alone in that mood.

Now I understand that being irritable and moody is one of the classic, textbook reaction to hunger and malnutrition.

One day when he came home from school I had just baked brownies. I took them out of the oven about the time he came in and the house was full of good smells.

Ten things parents can do to help prevent eating disorders in their children

by Linda Smolak and Michael P. Levine

1. Avoid conveying an attitude about yourself or your children which proclaims "I will like you more if you lose weight, eat less, wear a smaller size, eat only 'good' foods." Avoid negative statements about your own body and your own eating.

2. Educate yourself and your children about (a) the genetic basis of differences in body shapes and body weight; and (b) the nature and ugliness of prejudice. Be certain that your child understands that weight gain is a normal and necessary part of development, especially during puberty.

3. Practice taking people, especially females, seriously for what they say, feel, and do, not for how they look.

4. Scrutinize your child's school for things (posters, books, contest) which endorse the cultural ideal of thinness. Watch also for the failure of the school to include images of successful females in the curriculum. Without such images, girls are left with media definitions of thinness as a primary means of success for females.

5. Encourage children to ignore body shape as an indicator of anything about personality or value. Phrases like "fat slob," "pig out," and "thunder thighs" should be discouraged. It is noteworthy that being teased about body shape is associated with disturbed attitudes about eating.

6. Help your child develop interests and skills which will lead to success, personal expression, and fulfillment without emphasis on appearance.

7. Teach children (a) the dangers of trying to alter body shape through dieting; (b) the value of moderate exercise for health, strength, and stamina; and (c) the importance of eating a variety of nutritious foods. Avoid dichotomizing foods into "good/safe/lowfat vs bad/dangerous/fattening."

8. Encourage your children to be active and to enjoy what their bodies can do and feel like. Do not put your child on a diet

(continued on page 188)

Linda Smolak, PhD, and Michael P. Levine, PhD, are eating disorder specialists at Kenyon College, Gambier, Ohio. Reprinted with permission from the National Eating Disorders Organization Newsletter, Summer 1994.

Rick walked into the kitchen — and I'll never forget the expression of rage, frustration and despair in his face. "You baked brownies! How can you do this to me?"

That really hurt. I was trying to be a "good mother" and keep some goodies in the house. But he was right. Instead of helping him, I was tempting him with just the kind of non-nutritive food he didn't need. With our youngest son Mike it was easier. (Or was he more cooperative?) I fixed the same small nutrient-dense meals for all of us, no frills, no fat or sweets. He still ate almost nothing those two days before matches, but otherwise ate quite well.

One of the tough things about high school wrestling season is that it happens during both the Thanksgiving and Christmas holidays. I remember a friend with three boys wrestling who told me they hadn't had a Christmas dinner in 10 years that one of the boys didn't leave the table in tears, run upstairs and slam his bedroom door.

We normally celebrate with traditional holiday dinners, but I'd fill plates in the kitchen, spreading out the food so it looked like more, offer fewer choices to reduce temptations, and add big no-calorie gelatin salads. They weren't great meals and I knew Mike's thoughts were on the turkey in the kitchen, but we tried to make them fun.

Yet the night Mike won the State Championship at 105 pounds he probably should have had another 10 or 20 pounds just for strength and stamina — and his opponent was in much the same shape. It still hurts to look at that picture of Mike with his trophy.

Reassurance on size

It's natural for parents to want their children to be as perfect as possible, but when it comes to weight, "perfect" must be broadly and individually defined, advise two Iowa extension specialists, Carol Hans, RD, former Iowa State University Extension Nutritionist and Diane Nelson, Iowa State University Extension Communication Specialist.

In their public information brochure *A Parent's Guide to Children's Weight,* Hans and Nelson warn that children grow at different rates and may have very different body structures from their

Ten things *(continued from page 186)*

or exercise program unless a physician has verified that there truly are medical concerns associated with the child's weight (which is not very likely).

9. Limit how much television children watch. At least occasionally, watch with them and discuss the images of females presented. Do the same with fashion magazines.

10. Make family meals relaxed and friendly. Refrain from commenting on children's eating, resolving family conflicts at the table, and using food as either punishment or reward.[1]

What men can do
to help prevent eating disorders

Men have a special role in helping prevent eating disorders:

● **Take your role as a father, brother and/or uncle seriously.** Men play a very significant role in the emotional and psychosocial development of girls and boys. Abnegation of the role of father, in particular, in the name of work or success or lack of time is a contribution to (a) the emotional distress ("hunger") underlying eating disorders in females; and (b) feelings of powerlessness, insecurity and rage in males that fuel the oppression of women through objectification, pornography and other forms of violence.

● **Take personal and political action against sexism.** Men can contribute to the prevention of eating disorders by changing their own behavior and/or the behavior of others so as to:
(a) reverse discrimination against girls and women in school, in the workplace, on the streets, and at home;
(b) ensure that girls/women are free from harassment, sexual abuse, physical intimidation and other forms of violence to their bodies and souls;
(c) encourage girls/women (and boys/men) to accept and develop themselves as people, not as attractive packages based on restrictive ideals of beauty and self-restraint;
(d) develop relationships between (and images of) boys/men and girls/women based on respect, not exploitation.[2]

Reprinted with permission from "Ten things Men Can Do and Be to Help Prevent Eating Disorders," Michael P. Levine, NEDO Newsletter, 1994.

own brothers and sisters.[2]

To help children avoid future weight problems, prevention is the best cure.

"Ideally, parents help their children learn to recognize their own feelings of hunger and choose appropriate, nutritious foods to satisfy hunger. They also can help the child learn to see food as only one of many possible ways to celebrate a happy event, to ease disappointment, or to erase boredom."

And parents can refrain from comment about their children's size or shape, except in a reassuring way.

Hans and Nelson caution parents that a child who is too thin needs the same emotional support as one who is too heavy. A visit to a pediatrician can help put the child's size in perspective and provide a basis for reminding children that individuals grow at different rates.

However, when a child shows a sudden weight drop, other medical or emotional problems can be suspected. Professional help from a pediatrician, dietitian or child psychologist may be necessary.

Beyond reassuring the large child of parental love regardless of the child's weight, the appropriate parental action depends on whether only the child or the whole family has a weight problem.

If the whole family needs to change some eating and exercising habits, then the parent and child need to work together to initiate and plan those changes for everyone's benefit.

"For example, many social traditions are related to food and eating, such as giving food as a reward for completing a task, as a sympathetic gesture to ease hurt feelings, or as a cure for boredom," say Hans and Nelson. "These habits may lead the child to expect food in those situations, regardless of any feelings of hunger. By helping the child learn that such behavior is occasional, the child may avoid forming some of the dependent habits that can cause later weight problems."

If the child is the only family member with a weight problem, possible medical problems or emotional stresses need to be considered.

"Since a parent's primary role is to give support, any action that

Guidelines for approaching a person with an eating disorder

General guidelines

- Recognize your own attitude and amount of focus on your weight, body shape, and dieting practices. How might this be triggering or encouraging a friend, family member, or child to follow your pattern?

- Try not to use food as a socializing agent.

- Recognize that food has a purpose: to fulfill hunger.

- If there are family or friendship disagreements, try not to argue at the table. Such negative experiences become associated with eating and then food is thought of as a problem.

- Allow the eating disordered person to be in charge of their own eating.

- Avoid monitoring the food that the person eats, once the person is in treatment.

Guidelines for family members and friends

- Do not treat the person with an eating disorder like a child. If you are a parent, do not deny your daughter or son some parental guidance, but at the same time remember that he/she has many adult abilities which need to develop.

- When you speak to the person, speak with compassion and concern. Be as descriptive as possible.

- Avoid focusing on how the person looks with comments such as; "You're looking far too thin," or, "You're looking great!" This encourages body image obsessions. Instead focus on other areas of the person's life as much as possible.

- Explain what you suspect by describing the person's problematic behaviors. State your observations.

- Negotiate acceptable behavior with the person.

- Do not allow the dysfunctional behavior to be overlooked, otherwise, you are rewarding it. You need to increase the person's responsibility for his/her behavior.

- Set rules with the person regarding what is acceptable food to eat and how many meals a day are acceptable. Then focus conversations on other topics.

- If a person is binge eating, discuss with the person how you could help him/her.

- Do not use scare tactics. They are not appropriate and do not work.

- Give the person time to improve unless you suspect that his/her life is in danger. Negotiate a plan that may include certain behaviors such as eating regularly or decreasing purging. If the verbal contract is broken, seek professional help.

- If a person appears to be showing signs of extreme physical problems yet refuses help, a decision needs to be made by the parents and professionals to determine if treatment is necessary and how to initiate it.

- Try not to spy or interfere once the person with an eating disorder is in treatment.

- Provide specific information for help; names of treatment providers, phone numbers. There may be eating disorder specialists in your community or there may be support groups for eating disorders. Have the information available when you approach the person.

Guidelines regarding the person with an eating disorder

- The person with an eating disorder is sensitive to non-verbal behavior judging others' attitudes toward them by a fleeting expression, a tone of voice, or even the movement of your body.

- Try to remember their intense feelings of inadequacy. Attitudes of scorn, disgust, or impatience exhibited toward a person with an eating disorder intensifies his/her symptoms.

- Recognize that the person may deny your observations and be upset (especially if anorexic). Try not to be discouraged. Recognize that you have broken through his/her psychological defense. The person is frightened.

- Do not expect an immediate 100% recovery. As with any disorder, there will be a period of convalescence. There may be relapses. There will be difficult days when all of the old tensions flare up again.

Reprinted with permission from the National Eating Disorders Organization.[3]

denies support should be avoided," say Hans and Nelson. "For example, when a child is upset by playmates' teasing, a parent who responds with, 'When you get thinner they won't tease you anymore,' only reinforces the child's suspicion that there is indeed something wrong with him or her. A more positive response is for the parent to listen to the child express his or her feelings about that teasing, and then perhaps, ask if other children are getting teased and for what reason. This can lead to a discussion of: 'what do you think you can do about this situation?'

Parents should not treat the overweight child differently, such as giving the child different meals, desserts or snacks from the rest of the family, they point out. Similarly, putting the child on a weight loss diet is a form of punishment that asks them to ignore feelings of hunger and may lead them to believe there is truly something wrong with themselves for wanting to eat more than their parents want to give them.

Family coping

Parents who are concerned that a child may have eating problems should see their family doctor or an eating disorder specialist.

An adolescent may feel very uncomfortable talking about his or her eating, and may refuse to see a professional. Try negotiating, suggests Stephanie Fortin, MA, a Canadian eating disorder specialist writing in the National Eating Disorder Information Centre Bulletin.[3]

The basic idea is to negotiate slowly, one step at a time, rather than demanding that the teen enters treatment, while reassuring her of the concern for her health and well-being.

The National Eating Disorders Organization suggests the careful selection of a therapist, and advises patients, "You have the right to choose the gender of your therapist; you have the right to ask to talk with the therapist ahead of time to clarify his or her experience in this area and treatment approach. Listen to your feelings . . . If you feel you can work well with this person, then make a commitment to treatment."

NEDO offers reassurance that recovery can take time. "Working through an eating disorder is very difficult, an 'up and down' process." Relapse back to baseline or worse is a recognized pattern in eating disorder treatment, even after seemingly-successful treatment for one to three years.

Parents may need to examine their own feelings about weight and food, and work toward self-acceptance and size-acceptance. Modeling healthy behavior includes having nondiet foods and meals in the home, and using exercise for fun and fitness, not for appearance.

Once the child is in treatment, the parent should be there to talk with, keeping communication open, and sharing in supportive ways, says Fortin. Parents wonder whether they are too involved or not involved enough. They need to allow their eating-disordered teen grow up, to do the things others her age are doing. Giving advice and opinions in a respectful manner, as they would with another adult, will be helpful.

But parents need to recognize that they are not responsible for making the eating disordered patient well, she cautions. "The therapist will be responsible for that portion of the recovery process. This does not mean that you ignore the eating disorder altogether: Your support is important."

The therapist can help parents with coping strategies.

Don't let the eating disorder take over all of family life, Fortin advises. Focus on other interests you share. If family communication has broken down, family therapy may be needed.

Recovery may be slow, and parents should not be discouraged by good progress followed by a plateau. This is part of normal recovery. Even lapses may be expected. Recovery is hard work, so families need to celebrate small improvements.

Fortin offers these tips for parents:

- Learn as much as you can about eating disorders. You can be supportive by just understanding the issues your teen will be facing in therapy.
- Focus on issues of health and well-being. Avoid commenting on the person's weight or appearance. She/he is already overly focused on it.

- Understand the eating behavior as a problematic coping strategy for dealing with painful emotions and conflicts. Do not blame or shame the person.

- Encourage discussion around the person's current conflicts and concerns. Be prepared to help problem-solve and find supportive help from a professional.

- Be prepared to seek help and support for the entire family. This is a good way to develop mutually respectful coping strategies.

- Depending on family lifestyle, meals can be quite unstructured which under normal circumstances may be fine. Youth with eating disorders may benefit from structure and consistency. See meals as an opportunity for a relaxed time during which family members can catch up with each other's interests. Do not put undue focus on food, or force or withhold food.

- Avoid power struggles over food. Do not prepare or buy food for the adolescent and other food for the rest of the family.

- When the behavior of the eating-disordered person affects others, she/he is responsible. Bathrooms and kitchens should be left clean by everyone. Household or shared foods depleted by bingeing should be replaced by the person who binged.

- Take the adolescent to your doctor for medical evaluation if you are at all worried about her physical status. Signs of medical instability can be subtle, and might include dizziness, tingling sensations and "blacking out."

Following are exclusive writings by health professionals, working in the new paradigm, on how families can help children as they struggle with weight and eating problems and take steps in learning how to live and eat normally.

The new paradigm of trust

by Ellyn Satter, MS, RD

We are in the midst of a paradigm shift in our attitudes about obesity and the treatment of obesity.

The current paradigm assumes that all obesity is harmful and must be treated. Primary prevention is identifying individuals at risk and preventing them from becoming obese. This current paradigm is a control paradigm.

In contrast, the emerging paradigm assumption about fatness is that it may be normal for some people. Growing out of acceptance of size variation, primary prevention in the emerging paradigm becomes building positive feeding interactions and life style patterns that allow children to develop bodies that reflect their genetic endowment.

The emerging paradigm is a trust paradigm, based on observations that children have tendencies for a particular body build, including the food regulation processes and inclinations for movement that support those tendencies.[4] The task for the growing child is not to remain slim, but to maintain energy balance in response to variations in caloric density of the diet, activity level and growth.

The emerging paradigm of prevention is based on the hypothesis that children who are more grounded in their internal regulatory processes are less likely to make errors of energy balance, and thus more likely to sustain appropriate body weight regulation throughout life.

Parents' trust is prevention key

Within the trusting model of primary prevention, parents are supported in feeding and nurturing well. Fat (or potentially fat) children can be fed like other children when parents observe a division of responsibility in feeding. Parents take responsibility for providing wholesome and appealing food at predictable and pleasant times, then trust children to manage their own eating and decide how much to eat of what parents have made available. Primary prevention can also help parents raise an emotionally healthy fat child.

Fat children grow up to think less of themselves when their parents think less of them. Fat children and their parents need help in learning to deal with the prejudice and social and emotional challenges associated with obesity.

If a child gains too much weight, feeding dynamics, parenting, food selection and activity should be examined to detect what is interfering with the child's ability to regulate growth. The key question is, "What changed at the point that the child began gaining too much weight?" However, it is important to be wary of accepting currently popular explanations about cause.

The assumption in the control model is that children get fat because at some point they spontaneously begin to eat too much and exercise too little. Research shows otherwise. Fat children eat no more, or no differently, than thin children do. In fact, they are likely to eat less. Large-scale statistical correlations say watching too much television makes children fat but careful research trials do not support this finding.

Fat children seemingly move around less, but they carry more when they move and exert the same energy as thinner children. Children are ordinarily resilient regulators, and can accommodate to school-based shifts in activity and caloric density of food and still maintain stable macronutrient and calorie intake, activity and growth.

The emerging model is based on the belief that children have innate homeostatic mechanisms integrated with internal regulatory processes. Those mechanisms allow them to grow in a stable and predictable fashion and maintain genetically-appropriate body weight. The assumption is that children become unnaturally fat because some outside influence has undermined internal regulatory mechanisms and, thus, homeostasis.[5]

Research illustrates what happens when internal regulation is undermined. Children whose parents controlled their food intake were less able to adjust how much they ate in response to changes in energy density of food[6] Children followed longitudinally were fatter when they had feeding problems early on, and when their parents were preoccupied with keeping them from being fat.[7]

Abnormal fatness

The emerging paradigm definition of obesity is not fatness, per se, but fatness that is abnormal or unnecessary for the individual. Fatness can be normal for children who grow at the 95th percentile weight for height, or above, if they show a consistent and predictable pattern of growth, and any growth adjustments are gradual and occur over an extended time. If fatness is the result of unstable body weight with abrupt or acute weight gain, it is likely to be abnormal.

Children can get too fat when a parent or primary care provider systematically overfeeds them. Ordinarily, if a parent errs and overfeeds a child or the child errs and eats too much, the child compensates by eating less the next feeding or next day.

Children can get too fat when parents feed in a restrained fashion, hesitating to totally gratify children's appetites for fear they will get fat. These children lose their intinsic ability to regulate food intake and are prone to overeat when external controls are relaxed.

Children can get too fat when their emotional needs are not met, when they don't feel safe, and when there is stress in the family or in the environment. Among typical responses to these situations, children may overdemand food as a way of attracting the parents' attention or become underactive because they are despondent.

In all cases, rather than attempting to shift calorie balance with diet and exercise, it is essential to identify and resolve underlying causes in order to restore the child's normal regulatory and growth patterns. That outcome goal is achievement of the child's weight, not some externally defined (even modest) standard of weight. Striving for a particular body weight creates distortions with eating and feeding and interferes markedly with nurturing the child.

Does the new paradigm work?

Whether or not the emerging paradigm "works" depends on the outcome goal.

If the goal is to help children grow in a stable and consistent fashion and to achieve the adult body that is right for them, then, yes, the emerging paradigm works. What results from such humanistic and realistic strategies is normal growth. And normal growth works.

If the goal of preventive intervention with children's weight is the current one of keeping children from growing up fat, probably not. But the current paradigm proponents haven't kept children thin, either, even when they try harder. In fact, trying to externally control food intake and activity can undermine children's ability to maintain

California guidelines for parents of large kids

- Provide the child with lots of love and attention . . . don't pressure the child to lose weight.

- Have regular meals and snacks . . . try to discourage eating at other times.

- Let the child decide how much to eat . . . don't limit the amount of food a child can eat, or make a child "clean" the plate.

- Serve the same healthy food to all family members . . . don't put the child on a special low calorie diet.

- Have appealing snack foods available like popcorn, frozen fruit juice bars, string cheese, and frozen low-fat yogurt . . . don't have lots of high fat snack foods like chips, cake, pie, ice cream, cupcakes and doughnuts.

- Expect the child to grow into his/her weight . . . don't expect the child to lose weight.

- Encourage the child to be more active by playing with toys like balls, frisbees, jump ropes, and bicycles, by joining a sports team, by taking gymnastics, swimming, tennis or other lessons, by walking the family dog, or by joining a 4-H club, Girl Scout, or Boy Scout troop . . . don't let the child spend a lot of time watching TV or playing video games.

- Go on family outings that include hiking, swimming, and going to parks and playgrounds where everyone can play actively . . . don't let your family become "couch potatoes!"

From: If My Child Is Too Fat, What Should I Do About It? by Joanne P. Ikeda, University of California.[4]

energy balance and make them fatter than they otherwise would be.

Children have their own considerable capability with eating, activity and growth and the best approach is to support that capability rather than trying to outwit it. Working with rather than against these natural regulatory abilities enhances the likelihood of maintaining stable body weight throughout life.[8, 9]

Promoting size acceptance for children

by Joanne P. Ikeda, MA, RD

Families with children at high risk of obesity need extra time and attention from health professionals.

Most parents are very aware of the social stigma associated with being fat; many of them have experienced size discrimination first hand, and all of them have witnessed it. They are determined not to let this happen to their children. Often the steps they take to prevent obesity backfire on them.

One of the most common things parents do when they are afraid that a child is becoming fat, is to restrict the child's food intake. Recent research indicates that mothers who are more controlling of their children's food intake have children who show less ability to self-regulate energy intake, and as a consequence, may be at higher risk of obesity than children who are allowed to self-determine how much food they consume.[10]

Therapists working with children whose food intake is being restricted often find that these children are begging, scavenging, and even stealing food because of their fear of hunger. Parents attempting to exert control over a child's intake find themselves acting more like prison guards than nurturers and caregivers. Assuring parents that infants are born with the ability to self-regulate energy intake and that this ability needs to be fostered, rather than interfered with, is a key message health professionals must communicate.

In the early 1980's I conducted weight management programs

for adolescents, adapting Stuart and Ferguson's behavior modification approach for use with teenagers.[11, 12] Some of the youngsters I worked with lost weight, some maintained, and some gained.

All of them needed more love and acceptance. There was the large boned, aristocratic looking girl accompanied by a mother who wore a size 4 petite. "I hope you can do something with her, because I can't," said the mother haughtily. I felt like saying, "Sure, I'll just touch her with my magic wand and make her look just like you," but of course, I didn't.

There were the two bosom buddies; one was much fatter than the other. The larger girl kept worrying that her friend would lose weight, and thus have no need of their friendship. She made sure they visited the candy machine before and after every meeting.

The only adolescent who appeared to have escaped serious damage to his self-esteem was a big kid whose mother brought him in, saying, "Everyone in our family is big, so I don't expect him to lose weight. I just want him to learn some healthy habits."

"Yes, yes, yes!" was my enthusiastic response.

She was right, this boy was big. Big enough to intimidate any peers who wanted to make his size an issue. Plus he was good at using humor to help our group "lighten up," and even I was vulnerable to his charm. We needed his levity to ease the pain - the pain of knowing that your parents would love you more, your teachers would like you more, and your life would be wonderful if you could just look like the kids featured in *Sassy, Seventeen,* or *Young and Modern.*

I stopped working with fat youngsters when I realized that I was contributing to their distress by reinforcing the idea that there was something "wrong" with their bodies. But their pain remains with me. It sustains me and provides the motivation for my efforts to promote size acceptance in some very concrete ways.

Realistic size expectations

Health professionals need to help parents have realistic size expectations for their children. Children resemble biological relatives with respect to size and shape, and there is no way to "select" which relative a child will look like.

When a tall, large man and a short, fragile-looking woman have children, they may expect their daughters to resemble the mother, and sons, the father. But this may not be the case.

Parental dissatisfaction with their offsprings' sizes and/or shapes must be dealt with directly. Parents who are attempting to pressure children to lose weight by making their love conditional to the achievement of this goal, need to be told that they are harming, not helping, their children.

As explained in the University of California pamphlet *If My Child is Overweight, What should I do about it?*, "Being overweight may seem like the worst possible fate. However, it isn't. A worse fate is feeling rejected and unloved because one is overweight.

"You can made sure this does not happen to your child. Reassure your child that she will be loved by you always, whether she is thin or fat. Help your child to feel good about herself so that overweight is not compounded by low self-esteem. Remember, there is no reason your child cannot lead a happy, productive, full life at whatever size she turns out to be."

Parents need to understand that the primary environmental factor contributing to childhood obesity is not overeating; it is too little physical activity.

Most children spend more time viewing television than they do in school.[13] Instead of becoming preoccupied with how much a child is eating, parents need to make special efforts to see that the child has plenty of opportunities to be active.

This can include buying toys that promote active play, engaging children in active play, providing lessons that teach movement skills, supporting participation on sports teams, and integrating active play into family recreation. The emphasis should be on play - that is, activities that are fun and enjoyable rather than those which turn into imposed drudgery or fierce competition.

Bias-free schools

Because of their commitment to helping people, health professionals have a great deal of credibility with respect to influencing what happens in their communities. At community levels, the most important institutions in the lives of children are the schools. School administrators, teachers, and other staff can take an active role in establishing an environment that embraces and supports size diversity.

Children need to know that human beings come in a wide variety of sizes and shapes, and that there is no "ideal" or "perfect" body. They should be taught that every body is a good body, and that each person is responsible for taking care of his or her body. Most importantly, children should learn to respect the bodies of others even when they are quite different from their own.

These concepts can be integrated into almost every subject matter area taught in schools today.

Rules of behavior for both students and school staff can help to establish a bias-free school. Teasing, name calling, and put-downs or capping, should be actively discouraged. Very large or very small children and adults should not be singled out for negative attention, or excluded from activities because of their size.

There is no need to rehash the long litany of the ways in which our society discriminates against people who deviate too greatly from our standards for beauty. Even if we don't participate in it, we often stand by silently condoning it. Our children watch us and model their behavior after ours.

Going on a diet is an adult behavior that children willingly adopt. A perusal of the literature shows that children as young as seven report that they are dieting. If asked why, the response is, "So I don't get fat." By probing further, one finds that becoming fat is a very frightening thing to children because it means that you are "ugly, lazy, dirty, stupid and mean."

Fat has become the "bogeyman," the monster that terrorizes our children. Overdramatic? Only as dramatic as the newspaper headlines, "Too Fat Boy Murders Classmates who Teased him, Then Kills Self," "Girl drops Dead of Starvation - Afraid of Becoming too Fat," and "Girl Commits Suicide because Mom nagged her to Lose Weight." These are not from the *National Enquirer*. They are all articles I have clipped from California newspapers over the past couple of years.

Teachers and other staff may need to assess their own attitudes and behaviors about weight so they don't inadvertently model body dissatisfaction or promote size discrimination. The National Association to Advance Fat Acceptance has an excellent self-assessment pamphlet that can be used for this purpose.[14]

In the community

Communities need to value health and should demonstrate this value by supporting school nutrition, health education, physical education, and community recreation programs.

These programs are not "frills." They help children develop life-long commitments to physical well-being, health, and fitness through the adoption of healthy lifestyles. They are essential if there is to be a reduction in the prevalence of chronic diseases that debilitate so many people.

If communities don't foot the bill for these prevention programs now, future generations will pay much heftier bills for health care costs that are already a national burden.

Health care professionals are in a unique position to influence attitudes and opinions. Size discrimination is often practiced under the guise that it will motivate large children to change their eating and exercise habits so their bodies will become "normal," We must counter this by pointing out the flaws in this thinking. The primary factor in size and shape development is genetics, and children do not have any control over their genetic make-up. The second major factor in the development of obesity is an environment which fosters the [flowering] of this genetic predisposition.

Our children did not create this world where an overabundance of appealing, low-cost, high-fat foods are widely available at a moment's notice. A world where machines perform most of the task that used to require human energy expenditure.

A world where electronics entrance us into long hours of sedentary activity.

As adults, we must assume the responsibility for this situation and make every effort to change it. The problems are ours to deal with in ways that help, not punish our children.[15, 16]

Childhood obesity demands new approaches

by Ellyn Satter, MS, MSSW, RD

It is time for a new look at childhood obesity. Our current attitudes and approaches blame children and parents for a child's fatness and promise cures that we can't deliver. It's time to define the problem of juvenile obesity in a way it can be solved.

We have led parents to believe that children are too fat because they eat too much and that children can become slim if they eat less.

In so doing we set parents and children up for disappointment and unnecessary self blame. We have done the same to ourselves. In encouraging patients to try for weight loss, we find ourselves administering programs we don't totally believe in and accepting outcomes that leave us feeling discouraged and dishonest.

We don't know how to define childhood obesity, and have overreacted to normal fatness. Children grow through periods of fatness, but slim down as part of the natural growth process. Some children are genetically fat. It is possible that our interventions — restriction of food intake and subsequent struggles and preoccupation with eating — have exacerbated tendencies to fatness and interfered with a child's normal inclination to slim down.

Even when obesity does exist, we don't know what causes it. Fat children eat no more, or no differently, than thin children. Nor do we know how to cure it. Once established, weight patterns are extraordinarily difficult to reverse. Biological factors that function in defense of body weight appear to be extremely powerful. Even energetic, multifaceted weight loss programs with long term follow-up show only marginal success rates (if success is defined in terms of weight loss). It is estimated that most treatment regimens have very low success rates — ranging from 10 to 30 percent. While that is better than rates for adults, it is hardly a Cinderella story.

We can be honest with our patients about the difficulty of changing body weight. We can set aside weight loss as an outcome goal and instead focus our efforts on achievable goals: on treating the attitudes and behaviors that accompany the obesity — and predispose to it and exacerbate it. We can help our patients learn to eat and exercise in a healthful and positive way, to feel better about themselves, and to feel good about their bodies.

If we — and they — institute these changes, they might be thinner. But we can't count on it, and we must not promise it.

Identifying childhood obesity

The issue with identifying childhood obesity is — not to identify elevated levels of fatness — but to identify increased levels of fatness that are abnormal and unnecessary for a given child. It is to identify the child at risk and the parent who is concerned.

Some standards label a child as obese if his weight/height ratio exceeds the 90th or 95th percentile. However, the child whose ratio is elevated may simply be muscular or have particularly heavy bone structure. He may also be heavy because he is fat, but that doesn't necessarily mean there is a problem. If he has grown in a smooth and predictable fashion, it is likely that "fatness" or "heaviness" is normal for him.

Obesity may also be a transient growth phenomenon; children often go through periods of fatness. Most of them outgrow it.

Distorted growth

But if a child's growth is distorted — he shows a significant and prolonged increase in weight/height ratio — an environmental influence likely is distorting his normal growth process.

One of those influences can be a parent's over-concern about a child's eating and weight. Some parents are so fearful their child will get fat that they hesitate to totally gratify his appetite. Children fed in this restrained fashion become preoccupied with food and prone to overeat.[17] Parents may be concerned because they are obese themselves (the genetics of obesity make this a realistic concern), because they see themselves as maintaining an acceptable body weight only through constant vigilance, or simply because they live in our weight-obsessed society.

A child may also overeat because someone is systematically

overfeeding her[18] or because she is depressed or anxious and has learned to use food as a way of soothing her feelings. A child may under exercise because someone is overprotective, is intolerant of her noise and mess, or because she is depressed and lacks the energy to be active.[19]

Treatment

Rather than imposing food restriction and/or getting the child to exercise more, destabilizing influences must be identified and corrected. This will restore the child's normal regulatory and growth processes. Attempts to modify a child's eating and exercise patterns, and body weight, without correcting underlying causes only increases the pressure on the child in what may be an already-pressured situation.

Education on feeding management may correct the underlying cause of a child's energy imbalance. This must be focused on parents' feeding practices rather than on what and how much children eat.

Positive feeding demands a division of responsibility: Parents need to be primarily responsible for planning and procuring the family food supply, for maintaining the structure of meals and snacks and for limiting between-meal panhandling.

Given a feeding environment that is pleasant, supportive, and allows them the freedom to pick and choose from food that the parent has made available, children can take responsibility for deciding what and how much they will eat. It is when parents don't execute their feeding responsibilities or intrude on the child's prerogatives that feeding difficulties and disturbances of food regulation occur. Parents may fail to get a meal on the table, then try to control what and how much their child eats.

Chaotic parenting

However, at times, parents are unable to apply these principles. Some parents are so rigid and controlling, or so fearful of the child's obesity, that they can't give the child autonomy in the area of eating. Other parents are so chaotic, both internally and externally, that they can't bring order into feeding. At both extremes, families require referral to mental health professionals to correct the rigidity and/or chaos.

Frequently, these families will not participate in treatment and only want the child to be put on a diet. Such efforts should be avoided. It is absolutely unrealistic to expect the child to lose weight when the whole family system is set up to promote the opposite.

While dietary consultation about moderating the caloric density of the diet may be helpful, direct intervention with the child's eating is NOT an option. Putting a child on a weight reduction diet, or restricting food intake in even indirect ways (i.e., specifying "free" and "limited" foods) profoundly distorts the developmental needs of both parents and children. Children need to be nurtured. Parents need to nurture. Children need to be able to trust their internal processes.

Intervening with childhood obesity

Program goals

- Be realistic about outcome
- Allow the child to develop the weight that's right for him/her
- Maintain a positive feeding relationship — parent and child should *share* responsibility for eating
- Prevent overeating. (*Don't* promote undereating)
- Develop regular and reasonable exercise
- Support/enhance social functioning, including coping with a "handicapping condition"

Eating Management

Maintain structured meals and snacks

- Have meals and snacks at reliable times
- Limit *random* eating and (caloric) drinking between times

Maintain a division of responsibility in feeding

- Parents take primary responsibility for planning, procuring, preparing
- Let *even the fat child* decide

(continued on page 208)

Intervening *(continued from page 207)*

what and how much to eat from what has been provided

- Don't criticize how much the child eats or give the child "looks."

Help the child to detect and trust hunger, appetite and satiety

- Have pleasant eating times where the child can be relaxed
- Teach and model focused, mindful eating
- Expect reasonably civilized table manners — but be realistic
- Don't promote "stocking up" some times by restricting food other times
- Don't reward with food or use it for comfort — but do be supportive

Cut down on feeding cues (reminders)

- Confine most eating to the table
- Make most eating at either meal or snack time
- Put food out of sight to limit absent-minded eating
- Turn off the TV at eating times.

Keep the caloric density of food moderate

- Make moderate use of high fat, high sugar foods
- Don't deprive the child of such "treat" foods: that makes them more appealing

Think of the child as "normal" when making food decisions

- Plan and provide nutritious meals and snacks
- Make food selection decisions as you would for any child
- Trust your child's food regulation - don't fake it by serving low-calorie food

Use your own good judgement in setting feeding limits

- It is helpful to teach orderly, deliberate and satisfying eating
- It is helpful to be firm about structure with eating
- It is not helpful to deprive.

Look for causes if a child's growth changes

- Children's growth is ordinarily stable – if it changes, there has to be a *reason*[5]

CHILDREN AND TEENS IN WEIGHT CRISIS, 1995

Parents need to be able to relax and trust their children and those processes — not be police officers.

For children who are genetically obese (or who remain obese despite restoration of positive feeding and family dynamics), additional treatment strategies are in order. The goal for this child is to allow her to grow up to achieve a healthy body and feel good about that body and about herself.

Fat children can be physically active and successful in certain sports. Fat children can feel good about their eating, and have varied diets of high nutritional quality. And fat children can have good social and emotional skills. In fact, to be successful, fat children must acquire better-than-average social and emotional skills.

Obesity is a stigmatizing condition. Children who grow up with this condition, and their parents, need particular help in learning to deal with the prejudice and social and emotional challenges obesity presents.

Fat children grow up to think less of themselves only if their parents think less of them. Some parents are unaccepting and vehement about trying to change their children. Others blame themselves for their child's condition and are overprotective.

Fat children grow up to feel good about themselves if their families value them for their considerable worth, expect them to be capable, and see the obesity as only one of a range of characteristics.[20]

Prevention starts at birth

To the extent that it is an abnormal and unnecessary condition for the child, obesity can be prevented. This process starts at birth, with a positive feeding relationship between parent and child. Infants know how much they need to eat. They give cues to guide the feeding process and, to grow properly, must be supported in eating according to their internal regulatory processes of hunger, appetite and satiety.

For the parents of the obese child, an important part of prevention is helping them resist pressure to put their child on a weight reduction diet. Parents feel guilty and responsible when a child is too fat.

Their guilt is reinforced by health professionals, school, media, family and friends who think parents have "done something wrong" and expect them to remedy it. Parents don't benefit from criticism. They need help with their feelings, and support in pursuing a moderate approach.

Positive lifelong eating

Correction of factors that distort normal growth, and positive management of eating and exercise, should allow children to slow excessive weight gain and parallel the weight curve. If a child continues to gain at an accelerated rate, it is clear that underlying causes have NOT been resolved and further evaluation and treatment are in order.

Weight may level off and allow a child to rejoin an earlier, lower weight curve. However, trying for this outcome amounts to an attempt at weight loss that will distort the feeding relationship. Rather than trying for weight loss, we must measure outcome by the degree to which we have helped the parents and child establish positive eating and exercise behavior and functional social and emotional skills. Then we must let weight find its own level.

Of course, we can continue to hope that if families achieve these goals, children will grow up to be slim — or at least slimmer than they would be otherwise. The odds are good: Longitudinal studies on children and obesity show us that more children slim down than stay fat.

We can help children institute positive lifelong eating and exercise patterns and attitudes toward self and others. We can let them grow up to get the bodies that are right for them. But we can't make them lose weight. We can only do all we can — then we must let go of it.[21, 22]

Raising largely positive kids

by Carol Johnson

Big kids have a difficult time in our thin-obsessed society. Adults must send them enough positive, loving messages to counteract the negative ones they'll hear at school, the beach, at parties, and from the media.

As hard as it is to be a fat adult in America, it's even harder for fat kids. Adults are better able to sort fact from fiction and understand that weight is not a measure of self-worth. This is not as easy for kids who long to fit in and be accepted by their peers. Damage to self-esteem can begin at a very young age. If it's not mended, the scars can last a lifetime.

Building self-esteem at an early age is critical. Most adults with body image problems and poor self-images can trace the development of these feelings to painful events and messages they received as children and adolescents.

A local TV station recently did a series on overweight kids. While most of their obesity research was accurate (and I commend them for that), part of the series focused on a boy who had lost weight and now "felt better about himself." This sent a strong message that weight loss can improve a child's self-esteem.

I'm not opposed to weight loss. What troubles me is our inability to separate weight loss from self-esteem. Large kids should not be led to believe that losing weight will make them better people. Because despite their best efforts, not all kids will lose weight permanently.

Big kids have a difficult time in our thin-obsessed society. Adults must send them enough positive, loving messages to counteract the negative ones they'll hear at school, the beach, at parties, and from the media.

Some children may never be thin. This is not, by any means, the worst thing that could happen. Don't treat it as such. Just love and accept them unconditionally — and they'll have a head start on loving and accepting themselves.

It's imperative that parents and supportive adults provide larger kids with the tools to realize they're just as good as thinner kids, that weight is not a measure of their self-worth.

Here are some suggestions for bringing up largely positive kids:

■ Be sure your understanding of obesity is accurate and that you can separate myths from facts. This will help you to view a child's chubbiness as physiology, rather than a "defect."

■ Do NOT put a larger child on a diet. Most experts now agree this is one of the worst things done to overweight children.

■ Teach larger children that their self-worth has nothing to do with their weight. Emphasize their positive attributes and talents, and teach them that these are the things that have lasting value. Give frequent praise for talents, accomplishments and for just being who they are.

■ Be honest with larger children about remarks they are apt to encounter about their weight. Help them decide how they will respond. Tell them that many groups of people have suffered discrimination, and that larger people are one of those groups. Teach them that diversity of size is no different from diversity of culture — we must learn to respect both.

■ Be a good role model. Don't criticize your own body. If children see you appreciate your own body, they'll find it easier to like themselves.

■ Don't EVER suggest that a larger child's weight makes him/her less attractive or that no one will want to date them. This can cause lifelong damage to self-esteem. In a similar vein, teach them to respect themselves. A larger young girl may be thankful for any attention a boy gives her. Teach her that she deserves respect and affection and that anything less should not be tolerated.

■ Do make an extra effort to help your larger child find clothes that are in style.

■ Encourage physical activity. But let the child decide what activities he or she prefers. Don't force a larger little girl into a ballet class if she doesn't feel comfortable there. On the other hand, if she wants to twirl a baton, don't discourage her because of her size. Physical activity can be a family affair. Take a family walk every evening or set up a family badminton game. When I was a young adult, I went jogging with my dad. It was a nice time for both of us.[23,24]

CHAPTER 11

Prevention in schools

■

Schools reflect society's obsession with thinness and scorn for large people. The pressure, the harassment is all there — between students, between teachers, in the classrooms and in the halls.

Teachers tell me that they see girl after girl in the lunchroom choosing the salad bar over main-course meals, and coming out with only a small plate of lettuce. "I hope they are making up for it with healthy meals at home," one teacher said. Then she sighed — we both knew it wasn't happening at home, either.

This mini-world is an important and natural player in the effort for change. But parents and educators will need to recognize eating and weight problems more clearly, and to decide to approach them in a comprehensive way using new paradigm concepts which benefit all children and harms none.

Schools have long recognized the problem of hungry children. Many provide lunch and breakfast for kids who are neglected or whose families are poor.

This is just one step. Others are needed. It does not begin to touch the problems of kids hungry from self-starvation. And schools could do far more to address the role they play in children's lives when it comes to eating, socializing and developing self-esteem — qualities that aren't part of the curriculum but are nonetheless part of the learning process.

Adding the unified approach

"A student who is not healthy, who suffers from an undetected vision or hearing defect, or who is hungry, or who is impaired by drugs or alcohol, is not a student who will profit from the educational process," says Michael McGinnis, Director, Office of Disease Prevention and Health Promotion, USDHHS.[1]

Most schools already have prevention programs in place led by teams of teachers and other professionals that address six high risk behaviors: injuries from accidents, violence, suicide; tobacco use; alcohol and other drug use; poor nutrition; lack of physical activity; sexual behavior; sexually transmitted diseases and HIV, and unwanted pregnancies. Many also teach conflict resolution and how students can deal peacefully with anger.

But schools should also include and address body image, self-esteem and eating issues because they already relate to many of these high risk behaviors. Many children develop eating disorders in response to sexual abuse. Others smoke to lose weight. Low self-esteem can be expressed through violence, harassment and suicide, which also appear to be associated with dysfunctional eating and eating disorders. And the risk of preteen pregnancies increases as higher levels of body fat trigger early puberty.

Unfortunately, many prevention efforts aimed at reducing obesity or reducing eating disorders have been relatively unsuccessful in schools. Those who have initiated pilot programs are quick to point out that it's not been easy to show success. The challenge is to develop prevention programs that are both safe and effective.

Staff nutritionist

Of primary importance to incorporating these elements into schools is adding to staff a nutrition educator who has some special training in weight and eating issues. She may be a home economist, family and consumer teacher, or counselor with nutrition training.

In every school this nutrition educator would have the responsibility of training all teachers, especially elementary and physical education teachers. She would help them become aware of the issues and their own attitudes, and teach them to spot potential problems in students. Occasionally she could go into classrooms to present information, and to lead discussions and answer questions.

Teachers I've talked to say they'd appreciate this added dimension to their classes.

In addition, she would be a designated nutritionist for every team sport. In school athletics the risks are especially high for eating disorders, dangerous weight practices and steroid use. In the role of sports nutritionist, she would meet with athletes, coaches and parents at the beginning of each season, and be available to consult with athletes as needed. This is an urgent, immediate need, especially acute for wrestlers, gymnasts and female runners.

A sports nutritionist can help coaches understand their role in identifying and alleviating eating disorder patterns and obsessive behaviors, and teach them how to recognize early warning signs of disturbed eating.

This nutritionist can present or recommend special training programs for coaches and other teachers, in an awareness that many are caught up themselves in some of the same harmful behaviors as their students, related to dysfunctional eating, muscle building obsessions, and body image.

Finally, the staff nutritionist would be the school's referral person for students with disturbed eating and weight problems. She might meet with parents and form support groups for youngsters needing help, referring students with suspected eating disorders to specialists.

Working with a team of faculty, parents and community leaders she could initiate out-of-school events, integrating the school, home and community approach.

I'm convinced this kind of comprehensive program would reduce malnutrition, dysfunctional eating, eating disorders, and dangerous weight loss practices. And that it would also reduce the severe health problems, permanent injury and deaths which result from these high-risk behaviors among students.

Finding a way to help

Schools can help students develop the foundation of a healthy lifestyle that includes normal eating, healthy food choices, a positive self-esteem and balanced, active living.

Knowing how to chose healthy foods is a fundamental part of a healthy lifestyle. Kids should begin learning about normal eating in kindergarten and practice these skills every day. Cirriculums need to expand in every grade to deal with the level of dysfunctional eating, overweight and size prejudice that are real issues for students today. Teachers should be taught to recognize eating problems and dangerous weight loss practices.

At junior high and high school levels, classes in nutrition, child development and family living should be required. Students need to incorporate the healthy living, healthy family concepts from these fields into their lives in order to make a difference in improving health for all Americans in the future.

For many schools these classes and nutrition educators have seemed a place to cut expenses in these days of tight budgets. But they're criticial in improving student health. Administrators and parents need to recognize how fundamental they are to healthy family living. Concerned parents need to insist their schools offer these classes and that their own youngsters take them.

This is truly a health emergency and we must treat it that way.

Everywhere I go now people tell their terrible stories with haunted eyes: a sister who doesn't eat; a boy who hung himself before school started in the fall because he was overweight; a lovely granddaughter, 16, hospitalized in long term care for her anorexia; a step-daughter who "lives on coffee and cigarettes."

Teachers are hearing these same stories and watching them being played out every day in their classrooms.

Anti-smoking programs in the schools also need to incorporate information and messages on the relationship of smoking to weight. At the NIH workshop for Public Education on Weight and Obesity, Bonnie Spring, PhD, of Chicago Medical School, suggested targeting teenage girls with messages that educate them about the small effect of smoking on weight-suppression, minimize excessive concern with weight related to stopping smoking, and emphasize the higher health risks of smoking versus lower risks of weight gain.

Team conferences

Training conferences for health teams offer an excellent opportunity to begin effective programs to prevent eating and weight problems. Many states bring these teams together for annual training and program planning.

Last summer I had the privilege of presenting awareness seminars at both the North Dakota Roughrider Health Conference and the Wisconsin Wellness Conference and found teachers interested and concerned in these issues.

Linda Johnson, M.S., Assistant Director of School Health in N.D., who organizes the conference along with another co-planner from the health department, believes in wellness for teachers as well as building strong coalition teams. Her approach combines personal wellness skills for participants, along with the training and motivation needed to improve school and community health programs.

This approach and the unique collaboration between the two state departments of education and health have made the annual week-long Roughrider Conference a model for other states. Team coalition members include teachers, counselors, administrators, nurses, parents and school board members.

"We in North Dakota consider every teacher a health teacher, both because they are a personal role model and because anyone who reaches into the lives of children has the opportunity to be a health teacher," explains Johnson.

Teams return home enthusiastic and ready to work on the year's four short-term goals, which will further the longterm action plans they have developed.

Activities good for a lifetime

Many schools are well on their way to improving physical education so it focuses more on helping all youngsters be physically active in ways that will last a lifetime. There is more emphasis on being personally involved, less on winning games, grooming star athletes and spectator sports.

Good things are happening for girls in sports and athletics. In the two decades since Title IX, mandating full equality for women's athletics in school, the percentage of girls in sports has grown from 4 percent to 42 percent. And 27 percent of high school girls play on sports teams run outside the school.

Both girls and boys benefit from activity. But most schools need to increase the class time and improve the quality of physical education. PE should provide both training in lifetime skills, and the daily exercise needed by today's youngsters, who are often inactive outside school.

Healthy People 2000, which lists the nation's health goals, calls for daily physical education for all students. Yet, at the baseline set in the mid-1980s, just 36 percent of schools offered daily PE, and the number has dropped since due to budget cutting. Schools should also strive for more students to be active during PE. The Healthy People 2000 objective is to have 50 percent of class time spent actively.

Physical education has often focused on the most athletic students. Today it is seen as even more urgent to help physically underdeveloped children, since these are the most likely to lead sedentary lives. The less fit are the very youngsters who need activity most. They need special help in keeping motivated and in finding success and pleasure in physical activity. The President's Council on Physical Fitness and Sports identifies this as "the most urgent task facing physical education and other youth programs." The Council recommends fitness testing and remedial programs for students who don't meet standards.

However, this is done it must recognize the need to avoid stigmatizing or humiliating the less fit youngsters.

Classes should require daily aerobic exercise for students from kindergarten through high school, with a focus on fun and creativity, not competition. Competition isolates and discriminates against the less fit and larger children and discourages them from being active.

Additionally, many experts are calling for more after school participation in intramural sports, rather than focusing the school's resources on a single "A" team backed up by "B" and "C" squads.

More kids get to play on these teams which aren't focused on winning games and glory for the school. Communities that support intramural sports find it may be difficult to compete for time, gymnasiums and coaching staff, but that children in intramural sports often have more fun. Good athletes can benefit, too, in a system that frees up their time for other interests and activities.

Curbing abuses

For sports in which weight is important for peak performance, it is essential that coaches, parents and athletes keep a healthy perspective. Full nutrition and healthy growth and development for the athlete cannot be compromised.

Training while dehydrated is an especially dangerous practice which needs to be stopped.

Wisconsin is a leader in working to solve wrestling's inherent weight problems. The new program has proven so successful in relieving the pressure on students to cut weight, that it has seen a large increase in student participation and become a model for other states. Unfortunately, schools in some other places have chosen to drop the wrestling program rather than make needed improvements.

Wisconsin rules now require a minimum wrestling weight of 7 percent body fat for males and 12 percent for females, based on skinfold measurements by trained certified measurers. A 3 percent weight allowance is permitted. Thus, if a wrestler's predicted weight is 115 pounds, he will be encouraged to wrestle at 119 pounds, but could wrestle at 112. A wrestler is not allowed to wrestle in a weight class for which he would need to lose more than three pounds a week from the original date of his measurement. The allowance for growth during the season is reinstated, with two additional pounds allowed for each weight class on Dec. 25, and another pound on Feb. 1.

Healthy eating practices are now expected and actively integrated into the training program. A nutritionist works with wrestlers, coaches and parents.

Although reluctant at first, coaches now overwhelmingly support the new program, says Don Herrmann, associate director of the Wisconsin Interscholastic Athletic Association.

"Probably 60 percent of wrestling coaches openly opposed this in the early stages. They said we didn't need it, that skinfold measures aren't accurate enough, and it would bring too much attention to wrestling weight concerns. There's been a dramatic swing in acceptance. Now 97 to 98 percent are in favor of it."

He says coaches of other sports now want to be included in similar programs.[2]

Project SPARK

An example of a restructured elementary school physical education curriculum so it meets these needs is Project SPARK (Sports Play and Active Recreation for Kids). It's an ongoing research project funded by the National Institute of Health's National Heart, Lung and Blood Institute. Project SPARK places more importance on physical fitness activities such as swimming, biking, walking and aerobics, activities that can be enjoyed over a lifetime, and less on team sports as taught in schools today. Kids play games with the frisbee, jump rope on a regular basis, and take aerobic dancing classes.

Fifth grade teacher Julie Harris of the Turtleback Elementary School in Rancho Bernardo, Calif., has spent five years teaching Project SPARK and feels confident and enthusiastic about teaching physical education to her students. She credits SPARK's success to its researchers who identified several important factors:

- The importance of training and development of teachers. They also realize that follow-up is essential, says Harris. During the first year, Project SPARK trainers schedule a half-day refresher course for elementary teachers every four months. And once a week, a consultant is sent out to see how elementary teachers are doing and to assist them.
- A specific curriculum. The program is broken down into four-week teaching units, with each unit centered around a specific sport. Skills learned in the first unit can be transferred from sport to sport.

"More kids are more active, and even non-athletic students learn skills and achieve a measure of success," reports Harris.

"We want to create a model grade school PE program that will help instill lifelong exercise habits," says the project leader, James Sallis. "Because we want to connect physical activity to the rest of children's lives, there is a weekly class on how to develop activity routines outside the classroom. And it includes homework — just as in math classes."

But Sallis concedes that getting children to exercise after school has been more difficult than anticipated.[3]

In a nutshell, Sallis recommends that children and adolescents need to:

- spend some time each day involved in physical activity (games, sports, recreational activities such as walking to and from school or raking leaves); and
- engage in vigorous exercise at least three times a week for half an hour.[4]

SPARK energizes Navajo kids

Project SPARK was initiated in late 1994 as a preventive program in 12 schools on the Navajo reservation in the Fort Defiance area, near Window Rock, of Arizona. Approximately 1,250 children in grades three through six are involved.

Project SPARK is integrated into the core curriculum, and grade school students now spend at least 30 minutes, three times a week in moderate to vigorous activity.

The program has also been adapted to fit the cultural needs of Navajo children. Native dances are taught in the aerobics unit. Project SPARK's 30-minute program is divided into two sections: the first 15 minutes is spent on teaching aerobic skills, and the second 15 minutes on sports skills.

Project leaders hope this program will make a difference in the high prevalence of overweight among these children. About 27 percent of Navajo children are overweight, and 12 percent severely overweight, according to Paul Rosengard, a physical fitness specialist with Project SPARK.

"A sedentary lifestyle, a lack of facilities in which to exercise, and a diet high in fat foods coupled with a large number of fast food restaurants on the reservation conspire to make it very difficult for both Navajo children and adults to maintain a healthy weight," says Rosengard.

It's too early yet to know how Project SPARK will affect these Navajo youngsters' health habits, but he is optimistic. So far, teachers have been delighted with the program, and he notes that part of the success of any program is a teacher's enthusiasm.

"We want to turn the kids on to movement; and we want them to find activity fun and exciting," says Rosengard. "And I think that modest goal has already been achieved."[5]

Taking other steps

Any programs that schools develop to address the problems of weight, eating and self-esteem should be based on self-trust. Students need to trust their own body signals and needs. Students need to be liberated from false and narrow images based on appearance, and taught how to evaluate and combat media stereotypes. They need help in understanding that they can be healthy at the weight they are, and not focus on weight loss. Along with this, they need assurance of acceptance, regardless of size, shape or appearance. Programs with this new approach empower and strengthen all youngsters.

Progress should not be measured by a number on the scale, says Linda Omichinski, a registered dietitian and Canadian leader in the new perspective and nondiet movement. Her preventive program, *Teens & Diets: No Weigh*, is being used in several countries worldwide to help empower teens to effectively manage their own eating.

"For teens, a self reliant, health promotion model is well suited to the emerging and increasing need for independence and self concept building that is a normal developmental task of teenagers on the road to adulthood," says Omichinski.

Many prevention experts are saying the first priority for school-based programs should be modifying school lunches and making sure all students take physical education and that these classes do their job.

As they address overweight, teachers need to take care. Emphasizing obesity and its risks in preventive programs can easily increase fear of fat, thin mania, eating disorders, censure by health-care providers against persons with weight problems, social and economic discrimination, and the proliferation of hazardous weight loss methods.

Risk of intensifying existing problems is even more acute when in dealing with the vulnerability of children. The wrong kind of intervention is worse than excess weight, warns Ellyn Satter. She advises that any programs for overweight children need to consider and enhance psychosocial effects, and ensure that no child is stigmatized.

The branch of the National Institutes of Health which is charged with implementing the NIH Obesity Education Initiative in schools was expected to target large children for special obesity education and treatment when it convened a major school conference in 1992. But it was soon clear that educators were asking the National Heart, Lung and Blood Institute for a new approach.

Speakers noted that at least half of the adolescents who are dieting are not overweight. And even for large youth, the physiological and psychological hazards of dieting may outweigh the possible benefits.

They emphasized that it is increasingly important for schools and health professionals to provide sound health information and not simply follow traditional thinking. Dieting should not be recommended for adolescents, said one of the presenters, Pauline Powers, MD. There is need for public education programs to emphasize the acceptance of a range of normal body sizes and shapes.

"Food restriction decreases basal metabolic rate, decreases lean body mass and, with the almost inevitable regaining of weight, may increase total fat content compared to the period before eating," she warned.

Members of the group focusing on younger children at this conference expressed much concern about stigmatizing children at high risk for overweight in school prevention programs. If children at high risk are targeted, they warned, it will likely increase chronic dieting and eating disorders, as well as stigmatize large children. They recommended that no children be singled out for special efforts, but that all be targeted for the NHLBI Obesity Education Initiative. They also bluntly expressed their concern that many of the changes specialists were recommending at the conference focused less on increasing physical activity and more on restricting diet.

"Focus on how to make them healthier, as opposed to thinner, especially because making them thinner often does not make them healthy," they recommended.

Similarly, the group focusing on adolescents warned that NIH's national messages on obesity and weight may further stigmatize high-risk adolescents and lead to body image disturbances, eating disorders and decreased self-worth. They, too, recommended targeting all youth, not singling out those at high risk.

They further advised evaluating what is being taught on college campuses about the "Freshman 10," or 10 to 15 pound weight increase commonly experienced during the first year at college. Maybe it's a part of normal maturation and not detrimental, they warned.

Nebraska trial

Nebraska schools have taken on these problems. One of the most extensive obesity prevention programs has been the two-year intervention trial of nutrition and physical activity in third and fifth grades in two Nebraska elementary schools, an intervention and a control school.

Nutrition education was taught in 18 modules over two years by regular classroom teachers. School lunches were modified using "LUNCHPOWER!, Healthy School Lunches" program, and the exercise component was based on Physical Best, an American Alliance for Health, Physical Education, Recreation and Dance program. There were no increased costs or personnel to the school.

Nutrition improvements were considered moderately successful, both in teaching knowledge of healthy eating, and in changing to lower fat, lower sodium diets. However, the exercise component was less successful.[6]

Significant nutrition improvements were found over the two years during school lunches, and over the entire day's intake. In the school lunch itself, fat dropped from 44 to 28 percent, a savings of fat grams from 40g to 23g for the school lunch meal. By contrast, there was no change for control group in fat, and a significant increase in sodium.

The modified lunches were well accepted and liked by students. The lunch program was easily adopted, and lunch menus were in compliance with the new guidelines within four months.

The biggest obstacles to change were not in school lunch, but in physical education as it exists in most schools. Not enough time was spent in class, students were inactive during class, and curriculums devoted to team sports made it difficult to change physical activity.

However, changes were made in time spent waiting around, and waiting to play in team sports. Aerobic activities which easily fit into students lifestyles were emphasized at the expense of competitive games. Strength activities promoted lean tissue development. Activities were designed for all youngsters to exercise their large muscle groups for 30 minutes, three days a week.

But results were not as good as hoped. Modest short-term changes were made during class periods, but the activity did not appear to carry over through the rest of the day. Yet extreme caution is suggested in interpreting this data as measurement was difficult and had many methodological flaws. Also, expectations may have been too high for only two years of a narrowly focused program.

No significant differences were found in weight or obesity, and the only improvement in metabolic fitness was higher HDL cholesterol (the "good" cholesterol) in the intervention than control children. After two years, students in both the control and intervention school had significantly greater weight and percent body fat than initially, with no differences between the two groups.

The Nebraska researchers report that most elementary children average only 25 minutes per week scheduled for physical activities. And they watch television 24 to 27 hours a week, suggesting that activity levels at home are also low.

Another school program that shows promise is the Kansas LEAN School Health Project, implemented in two pilot communities in 1992. It focuses on changing behavior through four components: improving school lunch; integrating a nutrition curriculum; modifying the physical education curriculum to allow for daily noncompetitive physical activity; and development of an active community coalition to support the school program and provide additional support activities in the community.

The Kansas LEAN Partners is a network of numerous agencies, commodity groups, media, and private industry. Active coalitions in the two communities provide fitness and other events such as community-wide, noncompetitive track meets, nature walks with senior citizens, lean meat cook-offs, and the availability of juice machines in schools. Early reports note that in an attitude change, students have come to view fitness as part of their family and community lives, not just a school activity.[7]

Sallis reviewed seven school-based cardiovascular risk reduction programs with interventions of seven weeks to five years and found some modest changes in body fat. But none of the programs made much effort to combine education and environmental change. Most did not include either physical education or school lunch modification or involve parents, and they did not emphasize behavioral skill training.

"Thus, they did not demonstrate the potential effectiveness of prevention programs for obesity that include most or all of the key components," Sallis reported.[8]

Further, they did not measure results in terms of disturbed eating or stigmatization of large students.

Combating size prejudice

A program to teach students about size bias, reduce size prejudice and the stigmatization of large students has been developed by the Council Against Size Discrimination, led by Nancy Summer, of Bearsville, N.Y., a leader in the size acceptance movement.

In her workshops for 6th to 9th grade girls, Summer begins by inviting students to "get all the negative things out of their systems that they think and say about fat people . . . 'What do you think when you see a person as fat as me? What words come to mind? You can be honest.'" Summer brings out the stereotypes and negative language, writing the words on a flip chart, countering the negative stereotypes with facts and personal stories.

"We cover a lot of ground in the workshops: everything from discrimination to health to sports to fashion magazines. But always I stress my basic message: bias against fat hurts people of all sizes

. . . I explain that it isn't just large kids and adults who are hurt by size discrimination. Everyone else is hurt, because as long as fat is hated, everyone will be afraid of becoming fat. Fear of fat makes everyone unhappy and dissatisfied with their bodies. And that makes us have lower self-esteem and less self-confidence. And sometimes it can lead to dangerous diets and eating disorders. I share a lot of personal stories and listen to theirs. Some of the stories I hear are sad and frightening."

An important part of her workshops are looking at models, classic art, and comparing fashion layouts from Vogue and Big Beautiful Woman, and discussing the difference between glamour and thinness. Summer says the girls usually think the larger models are the prettiest, "And I have to remind them that girls and women of all sizes are beautiful."

Summer also discusses healthy alternatives to dieting and weight obsession. She encourages kids of all sizes to fight size bias by speaking up every time they see it, explaining that fat kids need allies when they are being picked on. They discuss ways of doing this. "It isn't enough to just not laugh along with a joke. It's important that you say something, whether it's privately to the person being picked on, or publicly to the mean kids that what they are doing isn't okay."

For the larger girls in the workshops, she says it is often what they hear their friends and classmates say about how to fight size bias that matter most to them. She feels validated by responses such as these:

"I learned that it's not OK to pick on fat kids."

"I learned that I'm okay and that I can be pretty even though I'm fat."

"I learned that my father is okay and that his brothers shouldn't be mean to him. Please send me something I could show my father about this."

Preventing disturbed eating

Prevention efforts to stop dieting and disturbed eating patterns at earlier stages can do much to help prevent eating disorders. Eating disorders are complex disturbances, often with a history of traumatic events or abuse.

Nevertheless, evidence that at least some girls progress from less to more severe eating problems underscores the importance of recognizing and preventing the whole spectrum of eating disturbances, say Linda Estes, PhD, Marjorie Crago, PhD, and Catherine Shisslak, PhD, at the University of Arizona medical school.[9]

The Arizona researchers advise implementing these three levels of prevention efforts:

1. Universal. This approach targets an entire population group or the general public with a type of intervention considered desirable for everyone in the group.
2. Selective. This is aimed at high risk individuals or subgroups.
3. Indicated. This targets individuals who have detectable signs or symptoms of disorder, or subclinical eating disorder symptoms.

Prevention costs are lower and success rates higher at early stages than when disturbed eating has progressed to the clinical stage. At that point, patients are more difficult to treat, treatment takes longer, and the disorder is likely to be accompanied by more severe medical complications.

The Arizona authors are currently involved in an extensive multi-site study funded by the McKnight Foundation, which is expected to provide information on the progression of disturbed eating. The study will follow girls from 4th through 9th grade over a period of four years. The girls will be assessed annually on risk factors for weight and eating concerns related to eating disorders. Results will be used to develop intervention programs geared toward the three levels — universal, selective and indicated.

Most eating disorder prevention programs have produced mixed results, and are more likely to show increases in knowledge than in attitudes and behaviors.

An intervention which made an impact on behavior and attitudes at a Toronto ballet school is described by Niva Piran, PhD, of the Ontario Institute for Studies in Education. It was begun as the result of a high rate of disturbed eating and eating disorders in the school, about 1.67 new cases per year of anorexia or bulimia nervosa.

Piran met all 100 or so girls, age 12 to 18, in small focus groups several times annually and used the knowledge and experiences gained to guide action and systemic changes. Together they created a cycle of dialogue, reflection and action which made changes through a period of eight years. During this eight years of intervention there was just one case of anorexia and one of bulimia. Students who became preoccupied with shape, weight or food issues promptly requested help or were referred by staff for consultation and, if needed, counseling.

The percent of graduating students scoring high on eating disorder measures (EAT score) dropped from 48 to 17 percent, and those reporting binge eating decreased from 35 to 13 percent. Surveys showed decreases in body dissatisfaction, drive for thinness, and dieting and purging patterns. Despite continued pressures for thinness in ballet, the students displayed a healthier approach to their bodies and their eating patterns. They strongly demanded a safe and respectful treatment of their bodies by school staff and peers.

Based on the focus group information, Piran says she does not view cultural pressure for thinness as a separate social factor. "Rather, I conceive of it as a form of violation of women's ownership of their bodies and related to other expressions of this theme, such as: harassment, violence, silencing, deprecation or isolation."[10]

Finding ways to stop sexual harassment, bullying, stigmatization of individuals and violence in schools is also considered of critical importance in reducing eating disorders.

From an administrative view, another compelling reason to stop this behavior is, it's against the law and could result in lawsuits.

Issues strong by 5th grade

Most eating disorder prevention programs aimed at adolescents have failed to make changes. Many eating disorder specialists now believe they come too late, and must begin in elementary or even primary grades.

By junior high school, negative eating attitudes and behaviors are strongly ingrained, almost as a part of female teenage culture, they warn.

warn.

Introducing eating disorder prevention programs in high school is much too late. This results in increased awareness of signs, symptoms and side effects but has failed to change behavior, according to Margo Maine, PhD, Institute of Living, in Hartford, Conn. She says it is unfortunate that so much time has been wasted on this effort too late in the process.

Prevention efforts need to begin in middle elementary grades, according to research cited by Smolak and Levine. By then, their studies show 30 to 50 percent of American girls "feel too fat" and 20 to 40 percent are dieting. By 8th grade, over 50 percent of girls say they have dieted during the past year. By high school, 40 to 60 percent of girls feel overweight and are trying to lose weight. Further, these figures do not reflect the immense pressure felt for body dissatisfaction by other girls, who are not dieting.

These attitudes and behaviors are measurable in elementary school, but younger girls lack the dieting commitment of older girls. Their beliefs about the importance of thinness have not yet crystallized.

Smolak and Levine studied dieting attitudes and behavior in grades one through five and found that by the fifth grade, body shape is much more important than in the earlier grades. Therefore, they advise that for primary school children the focus be on healthy nutrition and body acceptance, not eating disorders.

What to do in elementary school

Children who are already dieting during elementary school may be at risk for developing eating disorders because of the mental and physical effects of calorie restriction and weight loss failures.

Dieting and their susceptibility to messages of thinness may be modifiable at this point. This is a time when children's social attitudes and beliefs can be changed, their thinness attitudes are still evolving, and it is likely that parents can and will prohibit extreme dieting, say Smolak and Levine.

Discussion of eating disorders should begin between fourth and sixth grade when puberty development becomes obvious. For girls even younger than age eleven, and certainly before junior high, "be-sixth grade when puberty development becomes obvious. For girls even younger than age eleven, and certainly before junior high, "before their self-esteem begins to plummet for other reasons," says eating disorder specialist Paula Levine.

Yet eating disorder specialists warn there is risk that explaining symptoms of disordered eating, such as vomiting and laxative use, may unintentionally promote them.

While 4th or 5th grade may be early enough for discussion of eating disorders in schools, it may not be early enough for parents.

Paula Levine speaks to parents of newborn infants in newborn classes about eating disorders, and believes this may have an important impact.

Goals for elementary school

Goals for child prevention programs should have these goals, say Smolak and Levine:

1. Acceptance of diverse body shapes. This should include discussion of the causes of body size and shape and of prejudice against heavy people, as well as information about body changes in puberty.
2. Understanding that body shape is not infinitely mutable.
3. Understanding proper nutrition, including the importance of dietary fat and risks of malnutrition.
4. Discussion of the negative effects of dieting as well as the lack of long-term positive effects.
5. Information on the positive effects of moderate exercise and the negative effects of excessive exercise.
6. Development of strategies to resist teasing, pressure to diet, propaganda about the importance of slenderness, etc.

Smolak and Levine offer the following principles in designing eating disorder prevention programs for elementary school.

■ Involve parents. Parental cooperation is needed to attain program goals. Possible family problems may be averted or improved. They include mothers who are dieting and worried about their own or their daughter's weight, teasing by family members, negative or detrimental parental control over family eating. It is helpful for parents to examine their own values about body fat, dietary fat and attractiveness. Some children diet even to dangerous levels because of the encouragement of parents.

■ Tailor materials to the children's level. Instead of expecting young children to draw conclusions about how they should behave, simple "rules" might be provided, such as "children should play outside for an hour or more daily, and limit television watching." Discussion on dieting might focus on the short-term effects such as hunger, crankiness, poor concentration and fatigue.

■ Provide new ways to classify, evaluate and interact with people. Relabeling might involve using characteristics ranging from reliability to kindness to assess a person's value. It is especially important for girls to find attributes other than attractiveness or body shape by which to judge themselves and their success, such as academic, personal or social labels, they recommend.

■ Focus on healthy nutrition and body acceptance. For third grade and younger the prevention programs should probably avoid presenting the symptoms of eating disorders and disordered eating. But parents and school staff need to know the indicators of eating problems and that such disorders can occur in younger children. (Recomm by Smolak and Levine)

Eating disorder specialists say it's especially important to teach students how to evaluate advertising and the editorial slant of magazines that carry this advertising. Educate students to be insulated against the messages on thinness in advertising and the media, they urge; encourage them to write letters to advertisers and boycott products which are offensively advertised.

CHAPTER 12

Healthy choices

■

Healthy choices nourish the mind, body and spirit. It's important to teach children how to make healthy choices in order to overcome or prevent the weight and eating problems that dampen the spirits of so many kids today.

So how do we create an atmosphere that makes healthy choices for youngsters easy and fun, and the natural way to live? It involves families, teachers, schools, health professionals and communities.

I like to follow the Canadian lead: "Enjoy eating well and being active. Feel good about yourself. Have fun with family and friends, and you'll feel on top of the world!" As the Canadian Vitality program says:

> Feeling good about yourself starts by accept-
> ing who you are and how you look. Healthy, good-
> looking bodies come in a variety of shapes and sizes.
> A good weight is a healthy weight, not necessarily a
> low weight, so don't let your self-worth be deter-
> mined by the bathroom scales. Think positive thoughts.
> Laugh a lot. Spend some time with people who have
> a positive attitude — the type who look at the cup as
> being half full, not half empty. Positive vibes are

contagious.

Eating well doesn't mean giving up the foods you love; it means choosing wisely from a variety of foods that you enjoy. Your overall pattern of eating can include foods high, moderate and low in fat. If you want to enjoy a higher-fat food, balance it with staying active and enjoying a wide variety of foods the rest of the day. Children acquire attitudes about food first and foremost at home. Positive attitudes develop when food preparation and mealtimes are pleasant and fun experiences. So take time to enjoy meals and snacks with your children.

Being active means enjoying physical activity and finding fun ways to be active every day of the year — at home, at work, within your community. Whether it's bowling, mowing the lawn or playing hopscotch with the kids, an active lifestyle pays off. Make fitness a family activity; go ice-skating at the local rink, take an after-dinner walk together. Plan an active living vacation — a weekend hike, cross-country ski holiday, a canoeing getaway.[1]

It's important that children make the connection between health and pleasure. We need to emphasize the positive, enjoyable aspects of a healthy lifestyle. We need to de-emphasize weight by encouraging them to eat well, be active and feel good about themselves.

Feeling good

We need to help kids appreciate their strengths, abilities and unique traits, no matter what their weight.

We can help them to take pride in themselves and their accomplishments, appreciate the strength and ability of their bodies.

Children need loving homes where they feel safe from violence or abuse, where parents take time to listen and offer the trust for children to make their own best decisions.

In the community, they need the support of caring neighbors and other adults and to enjoy their company and build caring relationships with them. They need to have useful roles and feel they are needed at home and in the community. Adults in the community have the responsibility to protect children from violent persons and sexual predators.

They need good schools that involve them in the classroom and in extra-curricular activities and sports. Schools should be safe and free from harassment, stigmatization, and violence, and provide a friendly environment for socialization with peers.

We can teach them to appreciate diversity and equality, to accept their bodies just as they are and to recognize that healthy bodies come in many sizes and shapes.

Children and teenagers come in all shapes and sizes. Some store body fat more easily than others on the same kinds and amounts of food. And that's okay. All bodies are good bodies, whether large or small. Each youngster is special, and we need to accept, respect and celebrate our differences and the ways others differ from us.

Most of us can be healthier through improved eating and physical activity. Yet some kids may not be able to change their size, shape or weight much, even though they eat well and live actively. Some will grow into their weight. But keeping a stable weight may be a healthier goal than trying to lose. Studies suggest that keeping a stable weight is much better than yo-yoing up and down. It's easier to prevent putting on those extra pounds than to lose them later.

How parents help

In their Iowa extension brochure *A parent's guide to children's weight,* Carol Hans and Diane Nelson warn that children grow at different rates and may have very different body structures from their own brothers and sisters.[2]

They offer seven suggestions how parents can help children develop good eating and weight habits.

1. Be enthusiastic about eating a variety of foods. Help children learn what foods are in the different food groups and why it's important to eat some of each group daily.
2. Introduce new foods gradually. Offer the child a small portion

but do not force the child to eat it. Tasting will come more readily as the food becomes more familiar.

3. Plan and provide regular meals and snacks for the family. Parents set a good example by practicing healthy eating habits themselves. Mealtime should involve pleasant conversation, not discussion of problems.

4. Serve realistic portions. The appropriate serving size depends on the child's age and size. One possible guideline is to offer one tablespoon of meat, fruit and vegetable per year of age up to age five. Physical activity and growth spurts also influence appetite. Plan meals to include some lower calorie food items that can be offered for second helpings.

5. Buy fewer high-calorie, low-nutrient foods. Encourage children to think of such foods as occasional treats, not regular fare. Involve children in planning, shopping, and label-reading.

6. Avoid making nagging comments about a child's weight. Children who are above or below their "right" weight need emotional support.

7. Encourage family involvement in regular physical activity. Set an example by walking or biking instead of driving, using stairs instead of the elevator, planning weekend hikes, or swimming outings, or simply walking around the block after dinner.

Normal eating

Families need to learn normal eating so their children can learn normal eating. Dieting moms and dads may have forgotten that they can eat moderately, to satisfy hunger and appetite, and yet not eat past the point of satiety.

At the same time many kids and their families no doubt are eating too much food and too much fat. This can cause unwanted weight gain. Americans love to eat, and we are demanding bigger servings, eating bigger meals, and perhaps eating faster.

We need to remind ourselves and our children that it is not pleasurable to eat more food than our bodies want or need. We'll feel better if we stop eating when we are satisfied. The key is to eat enough food to nourish and satisfy, but avoid overeating. At the same time, we can trust our bodies to balance out an occasional episode of overeating, such as a holiday meal, over a period of days.

All this is part of normal eating.

Again, normal eating is described in terms of self-trust, flexibility and responding to body signals, by Ellyn Satter, international specialist on childhood feeding, in her book *How to Get Your Kid to Eat . . . But Not Too Much.*[3]

> Normal eating is being able to eat when you are hungry and continue eating until you are satisfied. It is being able to choose food you like and eat it and truly get enough of it — not just stop eating because you think you should. Normal eating is being able to use some moderate constraint in your food selection to get the right food, but not being so restrictive that you miss out on pleasurable foods.
>
> Normal eating is giving yourself permission to eat sometimes because you are happy, sad or bored, or just because it feels good. Normal eating is three meals a day, most of the time, but it can also be choosing to munch along . . . Normal eating is trusting your body to make up for your mistakes in eating.
>
> In short, normal eating is flexible. It varies in response to your emotions, your schedule, your hunger, and your proximity to food.

Normal eating is mainly regulated by internal signals of hunger, appetite and satiety. We eat when we're hungry and stop when we're full. It also includes some eating for social reasons and for pleasure. This kind of eating increases energy, health and strength, rather than being aimed at reshaping the body. Normal eating enhances feelings of well-being and makes us feel good — not ashamed, guilty or stuffed. Those who eat normally don't spend much time thinking about food or hunger. Such thoughts are low key, on the "back burner" most of the day, except at mealtime. Normal eating promotes clear thinking, the ability to concentrate, mood stability and healthy relationships with family, friends and community. People who eat normally will not all be thin. They will exhibit a range of weights, as their normal weight is expressed through a variety of inherited and environmental factors.

Satter says it is essential for parents to maintain a positive feeding relationship throughout the growing up years, to allow kids to feel relaxed and comfortable about eating and in touch with their internal cues of hunger, appetite and satiety. Underfeeding interferes with this, just as surely as does urging a child to eat more than he or she wants.

Satter teaches a Golden Rule for Parenting with Food: "Parents are responsible for what is presented to eat and the manner in which it is presented. Children are responsible for how much and even whether they eat."

This means that parents should select and buy food for the family, put meals on the table, have meals and snacks at regular times, and serve the food in a positive and supportive fashion. They need to trust the child to decide which foods and how much of each the child will eat. This is the child's responsibility, Satter explains, and parents should not interfere with the eating process by urging, bribing, scolding or praising for eating. Let children eat like children and eat as much as they want. Allowing children to make their own decisions about food freely lets them respond appropriately to their internal cues of hunger and satiety.

Unfortunately, this natural division of responsibility is often violated by parents with rigid or restricting eating styles of their own, who try to take over their children's eating, who urge them to eat more, to clean their plates — or to stop eating before they are satisfied. Satter says this sets the stage for disruptive and disturbed eating patterns.

"Even the fat child is entitled to regulate the amount of food he eats." Satter says this is sometimes a hard point to get across to parents.

Children need to be encouraged to eat when they are hungry, eat foods they want, eat as much as they want, stop eating when they are satisfied but not stuffed, enjoy the food they eat, and eat at regular times during the day.

Mothers and fathers have three responsibilities in feeding children, advise Hans and Nelson:

■ Parents need to offer the child a variety of nutritious foods at regular intervals. Planned meals and snacks give the child regular sources of energy, help the child develop sensible eating patterns, and encourage positive food behavior in social situations.

■ Parents can help the child learn to identify and pay attention to feelings of hunger and fullness. This starts with learning to distinguish a baby's hungry cry from other cries. It means not forcing a toddler to eat one more bite. It means sometimes having second or third helpings of some items.

■ Parents can demonstrate a healthy lifestyle. Children learn by example and are likely to want to do what parents do, whether it is eating chips while watching television, or going bicycling after supper.

Eating well

Familiy meals eaten at home help to structure children's eating in healthy ways. In eating together, families gain a better sense of themselves and moral values are shared in a relaxed setting. Family meals

Parents are responsible for what is presented to eat and the manner in which it is presented.

Children are responsible for how much and even whether they eat.

ELLYN SATTER, RD, ACSW
HOW TO GET YOUR KID TO EAT
. . . BUT NOT TOO MUCH

promote better family communication when they can be a pleasant time of reassurance, laughter, sharing of the day's experiences — all this, yes, with the television turned off.

In family meals at home, children learn the pleasures of eating healthful, good tasting foods in variety, eating moderately, and being satisfied at the meal's end. Food choices eaten in family meals tend to be well balanced, nutrient-dense, flavorful and home-cooked, in contrast to the sameness of the "fast foods" and processed and pre-packaged foods that make up so much of kids' diets today.

When teens skip meals or families don't eat together they miss out on all this.

Healthy eating begins with nutritious food choices. Parents are most often responsible for buying and preparing food. But children need to learn about nutritious foods so they can make healthy choices at school, with friends, on trips, and as adults.

Eating well means choosing a balanced palate from a variety of foods and eating them in moderation. It means following an overall pattern of eating that emphasizes choosing more fruits and vegetables, whole grains, lower fat dairy products and leaner meats.

Healthy food choices help young people grow, develop, do well in school, and feel at their best.

Food pyramid

Good foods nourish the body and spirit. Eating is pleasurable, relaxing. We need to allow this and no longer allow children to be deprived of the innocent pleasure of eating by the guilt, confusion or dieting of adults.

The Food Guide Pyramid gives us an easy way to visualize the five food groups: breads and grains, fruits, vegetables, meat group, and milk products. Kids need to learn to use and trust the pyramid as a healthy guide.

Eating a variety of foods from all five food groups ensures that a young person will get the 50-plus essential nutrients needed for growth, energy and health. A balanced diet, which may be balanced over several days, provides enough quantity from each of the five food groups. Eating moderately avoids the extremes, such as eating too much quantity or too little, of eating too much or none at all of high-fat and high-sugar foods which may be favorites.

Nutrient-dense foods should be the foods selected most often from each of the five groups. They are high in nutrients and low in calories, fat and added sugars. Nutrient-dense foods are often high in bulk and fiber — like an apple, corn or beans. Others, like lowfat meats, pack a lot of nutrition into small size.

While emphasizing nutrient-dense foods, it should be remembered that there are no "good" foods, no "bad" foods — all can be part of healthy eating. Kids need to enjoy a variety of foods and should not eliminate foods they really want, as it can lead to feelings of deprivation and eating problems. Foods that are calorie-dense rather than nutrient-dense may be selected less often and in smaller quantity.

The 1995 Dietary Guidelines for Americans give this sound advice for healthful eating:

- Eat a variety of foods

- Balance the food you eat with physical activity — maintain or improve your weight.

- Choose a diet with plenty of grain products, vegetables and fruits

- Choose a diet low in fat, saturated fat, and cholesterol

- Choose a diet moderate in sugars

- Choose a diet moderate in salt and sodium

- If you drink alcoholic beverages, do so in moderation

Kids who are afraid of certain foods avoid them at the risk of malnutrition. They need to learn that eating those foods in moderation is safe, and in fact is necessary for good health.

Most American teenagers need to improve their diets. Nearly all need to eat more fruits and vegetables, and in variety, to benefit from the wealth of important nutrients they provide.

The typical girl over age 11 needs to be drinking more milk —

Food Guide Pyramid
A Guide to Daily Food Choices

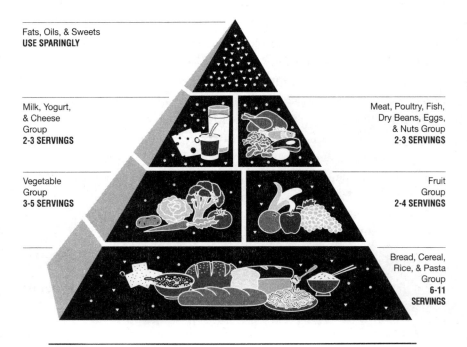

Fats, Oils, & Sweets
USE SPARINGLY

Milk, Yogurt,
& Cheese
Group
2-3 SERVINGS

Meat, Poultry, Fish,
Dry Beans, Eggs,
& Nuts Group
2-3 SERVINGS

Vegetable
Group
3-5 SERVINGS

Fruit
Group
2-4 SERVINGS

Bread, Cereal,
Rice, & Pasta
Group
**6-11
SERVINGS**

Use the Food Guide Pyramid to help you eat better every day. Start with plenty of breads, cereals, rice and pasta; vegetables; and fruits. Add two to three servings from the milk group (at least three for older children and teens) and two to three servings from the meat group. Each of these food groups provides some, but not all, of the nutrients you need. No one food group is more important than another — for good health you need them all. Go easy on fats, oils and sweets, the foods in the small tip of the Pyramid, foods which provide calories but few other nutrients.

Eating well focuses on balance, moderation and variety. Balanced food choices come from all five food groups. Eating moderately means eating enough for good nourishment, but not past the point of satiety, and choosing foods that balance out as moderately low in fat and sugars. Eating in variety from each food group ensures you'll get the many nutrients you need for health, energy and growth.

What counts as a serving?
Food Guide Pyramid

Grain products group (bread, cereal, rice and pasta)
- 1 slice of bread
- 1 ounce of ready-to-eat cereal
- 1/2 cup of cooked cereal, rice, or pasta

Vegetable group
- 1 cup of raw leafy vegetables
- 1/2 cup of other vegetables - cooked or chopped raw
- 3/4 cup of vegetable juice

Fruit group
- 1 medium apple, banana, orange
- 1/2 cup of chopped, cooked or canned fruit
- 3/4 cup of fruit juice

Milk group (milk, yogurt and cheese)
- 1 cup of milk or yogurt
- 1 1/2 ounces of natural cheese
- 2 ounces of processed cheese

Meat and beans group (meat, poultry, fish, eggs, dry beans, nuts)
- 2-3 ounces of cooked lean meat, poultry or fish
- 1/2 cup of cooked dry beans or 1 egg counts as 1 ounce of lean meat. Two tablespoons of peanut butter or 1/3 cup of nuts count as 1 ounce meat.

In using the pyramid, it is well to remember that the size of servings is a general guide. Smaller children will eat smaller servings; larger teenagers and older boys in a growth spurt may require more and larger servings. Even individuals of the same size differ in the amounts of food they choose and which satisfy their needs.

Children need to be encouraged to trust their bodies and respond to their natural signals of hunger, appetite and satiety, as they learn to make healthy food choices based on balance, moderation and variety.

at least three cups a day or its equivalent from the milk group, to ensure enough calcium for strong bones. Calcium is essential for healthy bones throughout life and is particularly important during the critical bone-building teenage years. Girls achieve most of their total bone mineral density by age 25. If they do not drink enough milk during adolescence, or if they are thin or often dieting and so lose bone mass, they may never develop the strong bones they will need later in life.

Children who are deficient in many nutrients due to lack of meat, poultry, fish and eggs, will benefit from restoring these foods in their diets. The Bogalusa Heart studies found that children who eat more meat are less likely to have deficiencies in important nutrients than those eating little or no meat.

Some teenagers have stopped eating meat out of fear it may be fattening, but there is no basis for this idea. Research suggests that protein, even in excess, is not stored as fat. Studies also show that meals with meat satisfy longer; one shows people who eat a meat casserole at lunch, versus a vegetable casserole, eat fewer calories in the next meal.

Eating disorder specialists and pediatricians are seeing alarming numbers of young children with stunted growth, fragile bones and stress fractures who have stopped eating meat and other animal products.

Some writers have promoted a low-meat Mediterranean diet as being "ideal" because of longevity in Italy and Greece. But others point out that on their high meat-and-dairy food diets, Swedish and Swiss people live even longer.

At this point, there is no basis for suggesting that lowering lean meat consumption has any benefits, certainly not for children, and it can result in severe deficiencies.

Robert Olson, MD, PhD, professor of pediatrics at the University of South Florida makes this point. He says, "The recommendation to modify the diets of children is without merit."[4]

Fat makes fat

All things being equal, calories from fat (chips, crackers, chocolate candy, pizza, ice cream, margarine, mayo) are stored as body fat much more easily than other calories.

Foods high in fat are often short on other nutrients and should be eaten less often and in smaller quantities.

The Dietary Guidelines advise reducing fat intake to 30 percent or less of total calories. This can be easy if we bring less fat into the house, add less fat in cooking, and use less fat at the table. Cutting down gradually usually works best. For example, using half as much table fat on the toast for a few months, then cutting that in half, and perhaps half again, can help a person change taste preferences without feeling deprived.

Many kids still have very high fat levels. However, surveys show most have cut down on the fat they eat.

Some have taken their fear of fat to the extreme, eating little or no fat. There is some concern that fat intake may fall too low; some experts are saying that lowfat diets are not appropriate for children.

"Good" foods, "bad" foods

When learning to make food choices, kids should know that there are no good foods, no bad foods. All foods fit well into a healthy eating plan.

There are no "junk foods," only "junk diets."

The idea that some foods are healthy and others unhealthy, suggesting that some foods can be used like medicine and others produce disease is false and unscientific, even though it is often promoted in the press, and even by health professionals who fail to understand nutrition.

While a balanced diet will usually be moderately low in fat and sugars, there's nothing wrong with eating high-fat, high-sugar foods in moderation, and in the context of an overall healthy food plan. However, these should be in balance, or children will fill up on foods that are nutrient-low, and not get the nutrients they need.

Living actively

Active living is widely accepted as a new, broader way of thinking about fitness. Active living is concerned with quality of life and total well-being, rather than excessive concern over body size.

Young children are the most active and physically fit of all Americans. They average one to two hours a day in moderate and vigorous physical activity. They are active because they want to be, not because it's good for them.

Unless we can bring about cultural changes, most will never be this active again. As children grow older, their activity falls off sharply, especially for girls after puberty.

We need to strengthen and extend the joy of activity that young children know, and help them carry it through into adulthood. We need to emphasize the sheer pleasure of being active, either alone or with friends.

After all, it's just for fun that 12-year-olds play softball all afternoon in a vacant lot. It's for the joy and exhilaration of it that skiers and hikers challenge a mountain. It's for the social and rhythmic, musical pleasure that young people dance nonstop three or four hours on a Saturday night.

In this new approach, everyone can succeed, explains Gail Johnston, a health and fitness consultant in Walnut Creek, Calif. It's not necessary to count heart rates, or calories burned, or work up to training levels, says Johnston. Nor is it necessary to lose weight to achieve the benefits of exercise.[5]

Benefits of exercise

"There are two main reasons why kids should exercise or pursue more physical activities: To be healthy as kids and to increase the probability that they will remain physically active as adults," says James Sallis of SPARK.[6]

Being physically active improves health in all sorts of ways. It lowers blood pressure, increases the "good" HDL cholesterol and increases bone density. It lowers stress and anxiety. Regular exercise lifts the mood of all teenagers, and is especially beneficial for those who are depressed or anxious. It relieves tension and helps put problems back in perspective.

The effect of exercise on bone density is particularly important during adolescence, because this is the time in life when bone mass peaks. Exercise also aids in distributing calcium into the bones.

"Think of the bones as muscles," Sallis suggests. "If you actively use or stress them, the bones will grow stronger."

Studies of tennis players show that the arm used most often, the "tennis" arm, for example, has much thicker and stronger bones than the "non-tennis" arm.

Being active may even make kids smarter. New brain research indicates that exercise is important in the development of intelligence. Studies find that developing the large muscles during adolescence helps to increase nerve connections for higher brain development.

Research also shows that students involved in sports do better in academics and are less likely to drop out of school, take drugs or get pregnant while in school.

Enhancing self-esteem

A recent study by Melpomene Institute and *Shape* magazine of girls age 11 to 17 found that girls who were physically active were more likely to have higher body image, a positive sense of self-satisfaction, higher perceived competence, and to say they like most things about themselves.

Being in athletics enhanced their self-esteem, and this was increased when combined with other after-school activities. In all cases the researchers found that girls who participated in a combination of after-school activities including athletics were more likely to have a higher sense of self than girls who participated in nonphysical activities or no activities at all.

Girls who were in six or more after-school activities including athletics were most likely to feel good about themselves.

The authors suggest that after-school activities offer girls a way to define themselves other than in terms of appearance. They allow girls to develop their interests, become committed and work with a group toward a common goal — all pursuits that are unrelated to appearance. An important finding is that nonphysical activities do not offer as many benefits as physical activities or a combination of activities. The interest and encouragement of parents in their activities also had a big impact on self-esteem measures.[7]

Activity recommendations

People of all ages are advised to engage in:
- moderate physical activity, accumulating 30 minutes during most days

For those wanting more benefits, add at least:
- vigorous activity for 20 minutes three days a week
- strength and flexibility exercise three days a week

Guidelines like these can be helpful in establishing a base. But Vitality suggests people shift the focus to being active in their own way, enjoying physical activities as part of their daily lifestyle.

Regular activity is extremely important in preventing obesity for both children and adults. Studies also show exercise is critical in reducing weight and maintaining weight loss over the long term. While these benefits may not show up as quickly as weight loss through diet, they are more lasting.

However, kids and their parents and coaches should avoid a weight loss focus in exercising. The intent should not be just to burn as many calories as possible so as to lose weight. This can be self-defeating and lead to dropping an exercise activity. So can keeping track of all the little dials on fitness equipment, which add up the calories supposedly burned, to determine how many pounds will be lost. This is not really the way it works and, anyway, individuals will differ widely in how much weight they may or many not lose through exercise.

The role of exercise in weight loss has often been exaggerated, bringing much disappointment and discouragement, warns Chester Zelasko, PhD, director of the Human Performance Laboratory at Buffalo State College in Buffalo, N.Y.[8]

Instead of focusing on exercise for losing weight, he says all people should exercise for the right reasons:

"To improve the cardiovascular system; to improve the strength, endurance and flexibility of the muscular system; to effect positive changes on other body systems such as the skeletal, digestive and immune system; and for other manifestations of improved health such as lower serum lipids and lower blood pressure — for the health of it!"

Less fit

Most physically underdeveloped youth can become fit if they are

---

Healthy People 2000

The Healthy People 2000 midcourse revisions call for increasing the percent of kids of all ages who take daily physical education classes in school. They urge that more time during these classes be spent actively, and that lifetime physical activities be stressed rather than competitive group sports. Lifetime activities are defined as those that may be readily carried into adulthood and generally need only one or two people, such as swimming, bicycling, jogging, dancing and racquet sports.

The Healthy People 2000 objectives, as revised in 1994, which affect children and teens are as follows:

- Increase the number of children in grades 1-12 who are in daily physical education classes to 75 percent *(from 36 percent in 1984-86).*

- Increase to at least 50 percent the amount of time in school physical education class that students are physically active, preferably in lifetime activities *(to 50 percent from 27 percent in 1983).*

- Increase to at least 30 percent the proportion of people aged 6 and older who engage regularly, preferably daily, in light to moderate physical activity for at least 30 minutes per day.

- Increase to at least 75 percent the proportion of children and adolescents aged 6 through 17 who engage in vigorous physical activity that promotes the development and maintenance of cardiorespiratory fitness 3 or more days per week for 20

(continued on page 250)

motivated at school, and if their parents understand the critical importance of exercise for each child's growth, performance and health.

Parents can also help by turning off the television and getting
involved in their children's chosen sports and activities.

While participating in school sports is important, those activities
don't automatically carry over into adulthood. Young athletes have
just as great a chance of becoming middle-aged couch potatoes as
their non-athletic buddies. In fact, a recent study Sallis conducted at

---

Healthy People 2000 *(continued from page 249)*

or more minutes per occasion. *(Baseline: 66 percent of youth
aged 10 through 17 in 1984. For adults increase from 12
percent to 20.)*

● Increase to at least 40 percent the proportion of people aged
6 and older who regularly perform physical activities that
enhance and maintain muscular strength, muscular endurance, and flexibility. *(Baseline unavailable)*

● Reduce to no more than 15 percent the proportion of people
aged 6 and older who engage in no leisure-time physical
activity. *(Especially targeted are blacks, Hispanics,
AmericanIndians/Alaska Natives, lower-income people, and
people with disabilities.)[2]*

Light to moderate physical activity requires sustained, rhythmic muscular movements, at least equal to sustained walking,
performed at less than 60 percent of maximum heart rate for
age. Examples are walking, swimming, cycling, dancing, gardening, yardwork, various home activities, games and other
childhood pursuits.

Vigorous physical activities are rhythmic, repetitive physical
activities that use large muscle groups at 60 percent of more of
maximum heart rate for age.

Maximum heart rate equals roughly 220 beats per minute
minus age. Vigorous activity is measured as a heart rate of over
60 percent of maximum; light to moderate is less than 60 percent.

San Diego State University showed the only difference between former high school athletes and non-athletes was that the former athletes watched more television sports shows than the non-athletes.

Encouraging girls

The roadblocks that still keep many girls from being active in sports need to be removed. More facilities need to be available for their use and more girls encouraged to use them.

For girls, the pleasure and health benefits of physical activity should be emphasized, not weight control. Looking to exercise for weight loss focuses attention on appearance, not ability or fitness.

Research shows that for teen girls who continue in sports, having fun is their primary motivator. Other motivators are gaining approval and respect, making their parents proud, feeling good about doing well, making friends and keeping in shape, according to Melpomene Institute, a Minneapolis-based group dedicated to physical activity for girls and women.[9]

Women's sports are still under-represented in the media, even though this is changing. Girls need to have more good female athlete role models. Also, it is important for them to see healthy female athletes of all sizes, not only unnaturally thin women in sports.

Changes are also needed in the way some journalists report on women athletes, exploiting and commenting on their femininity or appearance rather than their ability, strength and skill in the sport.

Obsessive exercise

Some teens take exercise to the extreme. They need to be taught that obsessive exercise brings its own problems and can take over their lives. They need to understand when to stop and how exercise fits into a balanced life.

Obsessive exercising is closely linked to eating disorders, and has many of the same features. A key to when exercise becomes a problem is often when the student's goals shift toward reshaping the body, from enjoyment or becoming fit and healthy. To help prevent this it is important for teachers and coaches to emphasize health-promoting goals, not weight loss or building muscles.

An obsession with the sport may be a "red flag" that an athlete is overtraining in unhealthy ways. Athletes at risk tend to talk and think about their sport constantly, often spending hours upon hours in the gym perfecting their workout at the expense of school activities, friendships and hobbies.[10]

Kids at risk can be helped more easily at an early stage of potentially abusive patterns.

Coaches need to be aware of warning signs of obsessive exercise and eating disorders in individual athletes. Experts are calling for mandatory training for coaches in how to prevent, watch for signs, and proceed in suspected cases.

Red flags for athletes

Nancy Thies Marshall chairs the USA Gymnastics's task force on eating disorders. The youngest member of the US gymnastics team at the 1972 Olympics, Marshall struggled with disordered eating.

She offers these "red flags" for athletes, coaches and parents to watch for:

- Obsession with the sport. At the expense of family, friends, hobbies and school activities, the athlete at risk tends to devote herself to her sport.
- Preoccupation with food and weight. Signs are thinking or talking often about food fat and calories, frequent weighing, skipping meals and binge eating. Motivation may be a belief that losing weight will improve performance or appeal to a judge's eye.
- Drinking an overabundance of fluids, in the effort to feel full.
- Laxative or diet pill use.
- Bathroom visits after meals. This may suggest the potentially fatal binge-purge cycle of vomiting food after eating.
- Wearing baggy clothing. Clothing may be used to hide weight loss.
- Dramatic weight loss.
- Physical deterioration. Malnutrition may cause chills, apathy, irritability, dry and pale skin, hair loss. Vomiting may cause callused finger, and sores on lips and tongue.
- Withdrawing from relationships. Feeling depressed, moody and

lonely.

- Overexercising. Compulsive exercise beyond her regular workouts may be a sign the athlete is trying to compensate for eating.
- Menstrual dysfunction. Missing periods or delaying menarche for too long (perhaps beyond age 17-19) raises concerns of premature osteoporosis and bone fractures (however, early menarche has its risks also such as for reproductive cancers).[11]

Bodysculpting

Athletic directors, coaches and parents need to be aware of the new media emphasis on muscle building and body sculpting. It is heavily promoted in new "muscle" magazines and advertising, strongly influencing some youth, especially teenage boys.

Strength or weight training helps increase strength, endurance and bone density. As such, it is an important part of many high school athletic programs.

However, weight training and body building can become detrimental when kids' goals become focused on reshaping their bodies for the sake of appearance. Coaches and trainers also may be caught up in their own muscle building to the extent that their influence may be harmful for youth.

The bodybuilding competitions and expert poses usually featured in muscle magazines do not focus on strength or skills. Rather, they are a form of modelling, showing off the appearance and muscularity of the body, for both men and women. Beyond having great size and bulk, muscles are clearly defined, rope-like, and veined with protruding blood vessels. Bodybuilders call it being "ripped" or "sliced."

This is competitive bodybuilding. It means there's almost no fat at the surface under the skin, and dehydration so severe the skin is thin as paper. Skin depleted of water makes the blood vessels stand out like veined leaves just under the surface. The technique combines intensive training, extremely lowfat diet, depleting fluids in the final days before a contest, and for some, use of drugs.

Education on the adverse effects is recommended.

Steroids and illegal prescription drugs are often used in bodybuilding. Steroid drug effects may be permanent and can put users at risk for heart disease and stroke. Reportedly they also can increase aggressive behavior and violence. Dependency is another risk of steroid use, according to Jim Wright, PhD, Health and Science editor of *Muscle & Fitness*.[12] He cites one study that suggests at least one-fourth of high school users of steroids are dependent on the drugs.

Exercise programs

In planning an individualized exercise program, Zelasko offers these recommendations for health professionals or parents.

• Emphasize consistency first. Since the goal is to maintain a lifetime of increased physical activity, it is most important to develop the exercise habit. Therefore, before recommending any in-depth, progressive fitness program, he suggests developing an easy, minimal workout and asking the person to develop a consistent pattern of following through.

• Encourage duration, intensity and frequency. Consistency is most important, but these are important in building fitness and improving health as the program progresses.

• Intermittent exercise is okay. If the person cannot sustain 10 or 20 minutes at one level, it is okay to break the sessions into segments of alternating low- or moderate-intensity work — this is interval training, used by athletes.

• Be a good example. Parents who want their children to gain the lifetime benefits of physical activity can be most helpful by modelling what lifetime activity means.

• Respect the large youngster. Everyone deserves respect no matter what his or her body weight. Nurturing is important. Maybe the child will lose weight or grow into the weight. Maybe not. But they can be healthier by exercising regularly and should be reassured of these benefits.

• Understand physical and emotional needs. It takes time to gain confidence in moving the body for kids who have been sedentary. If they are large, they may need to overcome shyness in using their body. As they become more successful in their ability to move, they enjoy it more and are more likely to continue. If using a fitness facility, it is important to find one where the emotional and physical needs of the child will be respected.

Parents can encourage more opportunities for community participation in sports and physical activity such as promoting safe biking
and hiking trails, swimming pools, basketball and tennis courts, and
local events and games.

CHAPTER 13

Changing to a
child-friendly culture

■

In a culture that attacks people for being different sizes, we must accept some of the responsibility for allowing the messages. And we must make changes.

If we want our children to grow up in families that love and talk to each other, we must work to provide them. If we want our children to grow up with solid, positive self-esteems and body images, we must work to encourage them. If we want girls to grow up free from sexual harassment, then we must stop it.

If we want the media to reflect to us images of healthy people in a variety of sizes, then we must work toward that.

If we want our children, who are afraid to eat or who overeat, to grow up eating normally and making healthy lifestyle choices, then we must also learn to support those choices.

Families, communities and schools

Changing culture is a huge task. Generations of people have molded today's society. Change won't be easy, nor will it happen overnight.

But in order to change our society into one that values healthy living, women, and many body sizes, we must enlist families, schools and communities.

There are signs that people are ready for a change.

The mood of the nation is swinging toward a yearning for stronger "family values," and safe and nurturing communities. Politicians on both sides are taking up the cause of strengthening the family and lessening the impact of destructive elements.

Worldwide, there is backlash against fashion's severe excesses in portraying malnutrition as glamourous, although the industry's resistance to change is nearly as strong.

When the Omega watch company decided to pull its ads from a British fashion magazine in protest against two extremely thin models, it received overwhelming support from the public and the media.

The Swiss watchmaker objected to *Vogue* magazine spreads that featured "skeletal" models Annie Morton and Trish Goff showing underwear and sportswear in body-revealing poses. Giles Rees, British marketing manager for Omega, complained the photos would encourage eating disorders in young women.

"It was irresponsible for a leading magazine, which should be setting an example, to select models of anorexic proportions," said Rees.

But Omega's chairman, Nicolas Hayek, reinstated the advertising. British *Vogue* arrogantly lauded the decision as a triumph.

"A complete victory!" crowed *Vogue* publisher Stephen Quinn. "It's good news in terms of editorial independence."

I hope Giles Rees will speak out again, and that he and others like him will follow their consciences in advertising. The more support they get from us, the public, the easier this will be.

Advertising and the media

Tackling the media — television, movies, books, magazines, newspapers, advertising, billboards, music — will be difficult. But the media carries destructive messages about body size, sexuality and women to all parts of our lives nearly everywhere in the world.

Regardless of difficulty, cultural changes can and must be made. Psychologist Mary Pipher in *Reviving Ophelia* says we can help girls fight cultural pressures by strengthening them, encourage their emotional toughness and self-protection, and to support and guide them.

"Most important, we can change our culture. We can work together to build a culture that is less complicated and more nurturing, less violent and sexualized and more growth-producing. Our daughters deserve a society in which all their gifts can be developed and appreciated."

She warns that it is critically important to change the way women are portrayed in the media, as expensive toys, the ultimate recreation, "half-clad and half-witted, often awaiting rescue by quick-thinking, fully clothed men . . ."

People concerned with these issues need to work together to change the focus of responsible media and advertising, and to deflate the poisonous influence of its irresponsible fringe.

The media needs to be encouraged to portray healthy lifestyles and healthy female images. I'd like to see a great outpouring of support for positive portrayals and a boycotting of the offensive.

I believe that if two or three leading teen magazines and women's magazines had the courage to depict girls and women of all sizes in their pages, the entire focus of the thin stereotype would change. Other editors, television producers, and Hollywood itself might be surprised to discover the beauty, charm and unique talents of real women in all their diversity.

The focus on malnourished bodies for women must be reversed. It is clear from several studies that fashion's ideal female is continuing to grow thinner. The incident at *Vogue* shows these pressures are increasing, not abating, as has been rumored.

Parents and consumer groups need to be vigilant in making bold complaints and leading boycotts against destructive stereotyping in magazines, television and advertising.

Boycotts can be extremely effective when marketed well.

A boycott of offensive advertising proved effective for a Boston-based consumer group that calls itself "BAM" (Boycott Anorexic Marketing). BAM forced the cancelation of Diet Sprite ads that depicted a bony, apathetic girl sipping a diet drink, boasting of her nickname "Skeleton."

BAM's boycott was picked up on national news reports and

Coca Cola hastily pulled the Diet Sprite ads.

Letters, phone calls and faxes, both of disagreement and support are effective in combatting destructive images. Targeting offensive advertisers is important, but their advertising mediums should not be let off easy; they are responsible for what they give the public. Producers and editors keep a wary eye on marketing and routinely slant articles to please their advertisers, often to the detriment of the public, as in the case of smoking. They can be urged or pressured to edit instead for public benefit.

On a more impulsive note, vigilantes are striking at offensive displays on billboards and buses by scrawling graffiti over thin women's bodies.

"I'm So Hungry," lamented the caption on one gaunt model.

"Please Give Me a Cheeseburger," another pleaded.

It is true that one person can make a difference, three or four working together can make a miracle. A nation motivated to action can bring about an attitude change overnight.

Female diversity

Girls need to be seeing healthier images of women and teenage girls in the media. Women need to be more widely seen as real people with diverse talents, of varied ages and shapes, deserving of respect regardless of their beauty or lack of it.

Today's beauty standards are so narrow that women in the media all seem to look alike — hollow-cheeked, passive, focused on their appearance, and extremely thin. They appear as decorative or sexual objects to be admired, used or discarded. It's a stereotype that sets 9-year-olds dieting and teaches adolescent girls that their developing bodies will never be good enough. It compels young girls to live as if they are being constantly watched, desired, judged.

Girls and women are not objects or toys, and it is most unfortunate when preadolescent girls are led to believe this is their role.

Teen magazines for girls need to change their editorial focus away from makeup, fashion, weight loss, and how to attract boys, topics of enormous interest to their advertisers. These magazines, or others which replace this irrelevance, need to include more articles on sports, careers, hobbies, and credible young women doing interesting things, so that girls are no longer led to "sacrifice their true selves" for the lookism issues they believe are uppermost in our culture.

As women move into decision-making positions in the media, I have hoped this situation would improve of itself. Unfortunately, despite the many advances made by women, this has not happened. Women's stereotyping in the media shows no signs of improving. It is time for women in these positions to make this needed shift.

As my contribution to furthering this change, we designate a day to honor women's diversity each year during Healthy Weight Week, the third week in January. On that Thursday, Women's Healthy Weight Day, we give awards to television networks, shows, magazines, advertisers and businesses that portray non-stereotypical women and confirm that beauty, health and strength come in all sizes. We've urged others to plan their own events for that day, and many do. Much to my delight, radio talk show hosts support and feature this event on their shows on that day.

Inoculate with education

Schools can do much to diffuse the power of advertising by training students in how to protect their self-concepts from narrow media stereotypes, beginning in preadolescence where media images have such powerful impact.

Even young children can understand the advertisers' self-interest in creating body dissatisfaction to sell products. Our children do not have to be pawns in this game. They can learn the pervasive technique of focusing on extremes to make products stand out: "if long legs are good, our models have longer and thinner legs; if wide spaced eyes and hollow cheeks are good, ours are spaced wider, our cheeks more gaunt than have ever been seen before." They can determine for themselves that these extreme images do not provide healthy role models for real youngsters who have real lives and interesting futures. Most of all, they will respond to clear messages that this is not acceptable with either adults or their peers.

Explaining the ease with which images are computerized today can make these models even less attractive and believable.

Consumer education for youngsters at all levels should include hands-on projects on how to evaluate television and print advertising of products they want, use or eat.

Girls, in particular, need to be helped to appraise skeptically all aspects of advertising, the dieting culture, and the language of advertising which encourages the belief that a woman's body always needs improving in one way or another. At this time we need training workshops in this.

Girls need help in recognizing how media images constrain not just their body shape, but their behavior.

Gail Huon, a psychologist at the University of South Wales in Sydney, Australia, writes in the journal *Eating Disorders* that girls must be taught to critically review the media images, articles and advertising not only for female thinness, but also for passiveness and submissiveness. They need to examine how women are portrayed in advertising as "property," and as waiting, receptive, ready to contribute to someone else's life. In doing this, they can reclaim their lives and see their real choices and options. Young women must be helped to respond positively to the challenges of their environment, in order to achieve their potential, she says.[1]

To combat the glamour of alcohol and drugs we also need to teach young people new ways to relax, to enjoy life and to cope with stress.

Protecting youth from abuse

Eating disorders and other disturbed and dysfunctional eating patterns often may begin as ways of coping with trauma, violence, sexual abuse, physical abuse, harassment, bullying and stigmatization. Communities, schools and families need to work together to protect our young people. Such violations of the self can have far-reaching effects which impact eating and weight in a variety of ways.

Youth who are singled out for special torment by their peers, or stigmatized because of their size, appearance, disability, homosexuality, or ethnicity deserve protection by the adults in their lives.

The National Education Association has declared itself ready to combat size prejudice in the schools. The largest teacher organization launched an investigation of size discrimination in the schools as a human and civil rights issue in 1993. The ensuing NEA report described the school experience as one of "ongoing prejudice, unnoticed discrimination, and almost constant harassment" for large students.

"This situation can be changed by education employees who are sensitive to America's obsession with the thin and intolerance toward the fat. They can foster a better learning and growing environment for students with unique needs due to size."

In 1994 NEA pledged to "continue to support efforts to foster an improved teaching and learning environment for colleagues and students who have special needs due to physical size; further, that NEA review its existing policies and recommend policy revisions in this regard, as appropriate."[2]

Unfortunately, most NEA members don't seem to know about this. When I ask teachers groups about it, I see blank faces.

Teachers and school personnel must take the initiative and move this policy forward in their local schools.

Sexual harassment

Sexual harassment is one of the important ways in which young girls' pleasure about their developing bodies is destroyed, experts say. It can alienate them from self, cause them to "hate" their bodies as a separate part of themselves, and oppress them with an overwhelming sense of shame.

Sexual harassment is seldom discussed, so girls bear their shame in secret. Boys, showing off for their peers, may not understand the harm they cause with cutting remarks.

For girls, consciousness-raising groups can be empowering. They are often surprised to find they have had common experiences with other girls that have little to do with what they believe are their personal inadequacies attracting these remarks.

In Toronto, Carla Rice and Vanessa Russell, Women's Studies specialists at the Ontario Institute for Studies in Education, organized support groups for girls on body image and body equity. They were asked to document gender oppression in the public schools, and to develop equity and health education programs for the Toronto Board of Education.[3]

In their early focus groups, they report, no one wanted to talk. Then one young woman would cautiously tell an incident she thought might be sexual harassment. Others declared the same thing had happened to them, "and then the stories flowed."

The girls felt relief when they found the courage to talk and realized they were not alone. They became outraged as they connected the shame about their bodies to incidents of violence and or harassment they had experienced. Each had endured her humiliation in secret, ashamed to tell anyone, because she feared she either deserved the belittling comments or had provoked them.

Rice and Russell watched the girls' shame turn to anger and their self-loathing to acceptance as they realized most other girls had the same experiences with harassment.

This shift from shame to anger may be a key to empowerment, they suggest. It's a transition from "I deserve to be violated," to "I have been violated," to "I do not deserve and will not tolerate violation."

As they shared their experiences, the girls grew more affirming and appreciative of each other, and became "a force to be reckoned with."

Can you imagine girls, their parents and teachers being a force to be reckoned with in this across the country? I can, and it would make a difference.

As a result of their work, Rice and Russell encourage wider discussion of these issues among educators and those who work with teenagers. They urge group programs to provide girls with hope, choice, and realistic strategies for resistance and change.

"We can offer young women some tools to fight against the weapons of oppression that have hurt them. These tools include giving them alternative images that celebrate women's nonconformity to the ideal, providing and sharing stories of resistance and empowerment, instilling a sense of pride in their bodies and themselves," they conclude.

Boys as well as girls need to be taught to recognize sexual harassment and know its consequences. Boys need to know what is not acceptable — so they don't go on to become the men whose firms are sued for sexual harassment and they can't understand why.

Both boys and girls need to know how to be loving and gentle.

It has been said that there are no rules in sexual behavior — until they are broken. This is true for young men as well as young women. When rules are broken, it's as if the offenders should have known all along what is acceptable, and they feel betrayed because they didn't know.

Young people also need to know that perpetrators will be held responsible for their actions. Potential abusers need to clearly understand the impact of what they do, to be taught ways to control their behavior, and to develop more appropriate behaviors.

This type of education may not fit easily into a society such as ours which flaunts sexuality and the availability of sex, yet has many taboos and fears about talking about sexuality and abusive sexual incidents. Yet it is imperative that ways be found to do this. Local decisions made with parents seems to be the best way to deal with this.

Prevention efforts must also address the cultural structures and messages that promote sexual exploitation and the manipulation of children's and women's bodies. Why do we still encourage beauty contests for little girls, teens and women, complete with swimsuit competitions? How can we allow these pageants to dictate, as they allegedly did to the 1996 Miss Universe, that a girl is too fat if she's 5-foot-7 and weighs 130 pounds? There must be other venues for showcasing the talents of these girls.

Preventing sexual abuse

It is the responsibility of adults — parents, teachers and institutional personnel, as well as potential perpetrators — to protect children from sexual harassment and abuses. This places the moral, ethical and legal responsibility where it should be, with the adults surrounding the child. When crimes are committed, it is the responsibility of law enforcement to separate the criminal from potential victims and to inform communities of convicted offenders in their midst. Both girls and boys need to be protected from sexually aggressive predators.

Civil rights groups may protest the need for anonymity. But I believe it is fair and just if youth are raised to know that the consequences of such action may be ostracism.

Kids need to be taught effective and safe ways of defending themselves against aggressors whether of the same age, older youth, or adults. But this shouldn't imply that children are responsible for preventing their own abuse.

Instead, parents, teachers, volunteers and administrative and other staff should all be educated in the detection, handling and reporting of child sexual abuse. Experts advise promoting public health messages like these:

- Sexual molestation of children is a crime.

- A child is unable to give consent.

- Sexual molestation of children involves an abuse of power and trust that is based upon coercion and intimidation.

- Sexual molestation is damaging to children.

- Preventing sexual abuse is the exclusive responsibility of adults.

Sexual abusers need to be stopped, and held accountable for their crimes. Offenders should be helped to understand the impact of their abusive behavior and to learn alternative behaviors which are more appropriate. In developing more effective treatment programs, drugs or surgery may be considered as well as behavior therapy.

Abuse may occur where it is least expected.

Stermac, Piran and Sheridan warn of incest. They recommend that first-time parents be targeted for intervention, informed about appropriate and inappropriate touching, and how to detect in oneself and one's mate the inclination toward inappropriate touching and what to do about it. They advise informing parents of the high incidence of sexual abuse within the family or by close relatives, and the tendency to deny abuse. And they should train themselves to build a protective environment for their children. Parents and designated school staff should discuss healthy sexuality with children and form an opportunity within this positive context to identify abnormal and destructive sexual situations.

"Young men need to be socialized in such a way that rape is as unthinkable to them as cannibalism," writes Pipher in *Reviving Ophelia.*[4]

Pipher points out that rape hurts everyone, not just its victims. It keeps all women in a state of fear about men, she says. Men are fearful for their women friends and aware that women are afraid of them.

But mostly rape damages young women. She quotes statistics that show 41 percent of rape victims expect to be raped again; 30 percent contemplate suicide; 31 percent go into therapy, and 82 percent say their lives are permanently changed.

Pipher points out that the incidence of rape is increasing because our culture's destructive messages about sexuality are increasing. "Sex is currently associated with violence, power, domination and status."

Health 'terrorism'

Parents are confused by the conflicting health and food messages in the media, and this is mirrored in their children.

The problem food changes weekly. Scare headlines warn of the risks of Mexican or Chinese food, popcorn, mad cow disease or alar treated apples. Foods are categorized as either valuable medicine or health hazards, labeled as "good" or "bad" foods. And after a brief flurry of stories the media moves on to other topics, leaving consumers shaken and more fearful than before.

The paradox is that this national panic comes at a time when Americans are healthier and living longer than ever before, and when the U.S. food supply is one of the safest and healthiest in the world.

In actual fact, many of these risks are negligible. If they make any difference at all, it may only be three or four days of longevity for a few individuals. Studies are often very preliminary, or represent one unorthodox view of an obscure controversy. Often the reports are meant for scientists talking to scientists, better discussed in a college lab than the front page of the daily newspaper. Headline-seekers and groups with a political agenda have learned how to manipulate the media.

Also, some of this fearmongering may be a deliberate way to lay a smoke screen over smoking issues, charges Elizabeth Whelan, president of the American Council on Science and Health.

She says the nearly $6 billion spent yearly by the tobacco industry on advertising and promotion, plus the deep roots the tobacco industry has forged throughout corporate America, and the financial support it gives members of Congress, that "clearly buys silence and diversion" to hide the fact that half of all premature deaths before age 80, a half million a year, are directly and causally related to tobacco. She says nothing could make "this killer advertiser more content than having the word 'carcinogen' used so often it loses all its meaning. Remember: When everything is dangerous, then nothing is."

"The leading cause of death has enough clout to keep the legislative and publicity spotlights off the cigarette — and on the multitude of nonrisks around us."

Stop fearmongering

Whelan calls on scientists, policy makers, the media and consumers to stop the fearmongering and implement changes such as the following:

- Emphasize that our food supply is safe. Keep reassuring the press and public of the truth: that America has the safest, healthiest, most enviable food supply in the world. The rarity of adverse incidents should be used to prove, rather than dispute, this fact.
- Return to mainstream science that defends reason and rationality. Whelan says many scientists don't want to get involved, and yet they must. And they must communicate, not in uncertainties as scientists are wont to do, but in easily understandable terms that make clear what the relative risks are.
- Emphasize healthy nutrition messages and insist on balance. Restore acceptance of the basic principle that health depends

on the total diet, not on a few special components. Convey the message that all foods can fit into a healthy diet. All the five food groups in variety — the meat and milk groups as well as fruits, vegetables and grains are important for healthy, balanced nutrition. Further, there are no "bad" foods. Even high-fat foods, the current bugaboo, can be balanced by low-fat foods in a diet that is 30 percent fat.

■ Diffuse the power of "health terrorists" and "food terrorists" to grab headlines, whether these are ill-informed consumer groups, journalists on a "politically correct" mission, talk show hosts seeking higher ratings, radical animal rights groups, or scientists shoring up their grant funding. Whelan calls these people spokesmen from the "Chicken Little School of Environmental Hyperbole." They need to be exposed as such, by insisting on balance, reason and a discussion of relative risks.

■ Expose the corruption of "politically correct science." This trendy ideology makes environmentalism and consumerism the new religion, says Whelan. It is against industry, technology, and free enterprise, and has abandoned science, reason and rationality. It is an ideology which has infused the press with false notions that American health is at risk from environmental pollution, additives, meat, and plants treated with harmless pesticides. There is no scientific evidence to suggest that any of these are health risks.

■ Reduce the influence of the tobacco industry to silence criticism and divert attention from the real health risks. When over 1,300 Americans die prematurely every day from tobacco, and some 300 die of the affects of alcohol every day, it is almost ludicrous that nonrisks get the major headlines. Tobacco has privileged status which needs to be stripped. It is time to stop smoking advertising in print media, as the billions of dollars spent on advertising have been effective in silencing most smoking criticism in magazines and newspapers.

Consumers need to tune out these "health terrorist" headlines. In my view, if a problem really exists, we'll hear about it soon enough. Meanwhile, we need to just overlook scaremongering mes-sages. It's a bit like my advice about the new weight loss miracles: "Wait two years, then you will know."

CHAPTER 14

Call to action

It's time to develop a vision and direction. This is an urgent challenge for America and many other countries throughout the world.

We need to deal with the current weight and eating crisis in healthy ways — ways that don't repeat the mistakes of the past.

The health promoting approach recognizes the interrelatedness of four major problems: dysfunctional eating, eating disorders, size prejudice, overweight. It furthers healthy growth and development of the whole child in mind, body and spirit, and it includes every child of every size.

The underlying unity of this approach is that what is healthy for the largest kid on the block is also healthy for the thinnest. All children need assurance of acceptance, regardless of size, shape or appearance. We need to help young people build self-esteem, learn assertiveness and healthy coping skills, and to develop their unique potential as lovable, capable, valuable individuals who take pride in themselves and appreciate diversity in others.

As in the Canadian *Vitality* program this new paradigm promotes eating well, living actively and feeling good about ourselves. This message needs to be communicated consistently within the health community, general public and the media.

The process of developing a unified vision needs to involve parents, teachers, doctors, nurses, policy makers and specialists in related areas — people of insight, intelligence and integrity. We can no longer permit these critical decisions to be made by persons who refuse to consider the potential effect of their decisions on children, women and minorities, or who serve the weight loss industry.

Challenges for wellness and wholeness

How can we promote wellness and wholeness in more positive ways for children and youth of all sizes? How can we reach a shared vision and effectively communicate that vision?

Challenges for change involve the five areas of attitude, lifestyle, prevention, health care, and knowledge.[1]

1. Attitude

As individuals and a nation we need to promote a shift in attitudes toward:

- A wider awareness and concern for the issues of weight and eating, and their interrelationships; their importance in children's healthy growth and development.
- Greater appreciation for healthy lifestyles and balanced, wholesome living. People need to feel encouraged to make healthy changes in their own lives. Focus on the pleasurable, energizing and healthful benefits, not on weight or body image.
- Less cultural concern for appearance, and more for values of character, responsibility, achievement, family and community. Convey to girls who are fixated on appearance as a way of belonging, that they will be nicer, more interesting people and have better lives when well nourished.
- More respect for individuals. A higher abhorrence of violations against persons, including mental, physical and sexual abuse, harassment and stigmatization.
- Acceptance of a wider range of sizes. Appreciation of diversity, that beauty comes in all shapes and sizes. Away from extreme thinness as the "ideal" body type.
- The media is a powerful instrument for attitude change. It is

needed to help promote healthy lifestyles that prevent weight and eating problems for children and adults. Expose the promotion of body dissatisfaction and the emphasis on appearance to sell products, and reduce negative impact through encouraging education, complaints and boycotting.

- The news media needs to more closely evaluate health news, consider the source, and put it in the perspective of how much risk there really is (compared to smoking, perhaps). Expose the source of "politically correct" views that may be unsound and detrimental to health and well-being, rather than perpetuating them.

- The media needs to help in promoting a stronger appreciation of diversity, rejecting the "bimbo mentality," and shifting toward portraying women as real people. Strong, capable, intelligent women need to be much more visible in the media and public life — talented, caring women who will be role models for our daughters and gain the respect of our sons.

2. Lifestyle

We need to promote healthy lifestyle changes which:

- Promote a physically active population. Improve physical education programs in schools and motivate youth to continue being active through life. A national public health program to encourage active living in the U.S., similar to that in many other countries, is long overdue.

- Encourage moderate, wholesome eating, a varied and balanced diet, moderately low in fat, avoiding extremes, based on normal eating patterns. Also eating as a pleasurable experience.

- Promote the attainment of genetically favorable weight for growing children, and natural, stable weights after mature height and size is reached. Stop ineffective, unsafe weight loss practices. Stop dieting.

- Improve stress levels. Find effective ways to reduce or manage stress more effectively. Enrich self-esteem, self-acceptance, feelings of being needed, and positive relations with family, friends, community. Focus on balance and moderation, and satisfaction with life. Avoid extremes.

■ Reduce violence, sexual abuse, harassment and stigmatization, particularly against children and young girls; find effective ways to protect girls from aggressive men. Provide more widespread victim counseling or programs that reach all who are abused. Increase law enforcement and incarceration to separate abusers from potential victims.

■ Promote environments that support being active, eating well and reducing stress through schools, health care providers, the community, media and home. Communities can do much to encourage active living: developing safe, well-lighted playgrounds, parks, swimming pools, skating rinks, and trails for walking, bicycling and cross-country skiing. They can open school gymnasiums to the public, provide recreation centers, and organize fitness campaigns and events. At the national level public health efforts should advocate the pleasures and health benefits of an active lifestyle, not weight loss, especially for children, adolescents, the elderly and lower socioeconomic populations.

3. Prevention

Prevention programs aimed at reducing weight and eating problems need to be launched nationwide. Yet there are grave concerns about advocating such programs prematurely, without adequate research into their safety and effectiveness. It is clear the wrong kind of programs can cause much harm. Guidelines for these programs may follow these steps:

■ Develop goals aimed at three levels: (1) the prevention of weight and eating problems for all youngsters, (2) identification of and possible intervention and support groups for youth with early potential problems, (3) referral of individuals with severe problems to specialists, while avoiding stigmatizing them.

■ Develop and pilot test prevention programs, including culture-specific programs for high-risk minority and ethnic groups. Evaluate results, and report benefits and any potentially harmful effects.

■ Fine-tune worthwhile and effective prevention programs and implement them in schools and communities. Continue to test and evaluate. Communities need to come together to support and nurture their youth, providing strong intergenerational relationships.

4. Health care

We need to promote a shift in both national policy and local health care services to:

■ Ensure that health care providers promote healthy lifestyles and being healthy at every size.

■ Focus on improving the health of large kids, not on weight loss. Stop submitting large children to diets, drugs, and weight loss surgery without proof of longterm safety and effectiveness; children have time to wait until proven methods are developed.

■ Reduce size prejudice in health care. Many health care providers need to become aware of and work to overcome their own biases, so that large people feel free to come to them for health care.

■ Identify and treat disturbed or disordered eating at an early stage; prevent eating disorders.

■ Improve access to qualified services for high risk populations.

■ Develop a sound policy on use of weight loss drugs. Require proof of longterm safety and effectiveness, not the brief one-year studies claimed adequate today. Begin dialogue on ethical use of drugs. When weight loss drugs become effective, will it be ethical to prescribe them widely throughout the population, for children as well as adults? What are the advantages and disadvantages? Today's promotion of longterm drug treatment for obesity by many health care providers and their insistance that insurance pay for this is a cause for concern — the potential for abuse now and in the future is high. Many federal and academic specialists warn there is "insufficient research," on longterm effects.[2]

■ Require medical students to study basic nutrition. Expand medical training to include overweight and eating disorders, as well as promoting more reliance on these specialists and refering patients to specialists in these areas.

■ Regulate the weight loss industry, as any other health-related business. Require adequate safety and effectiveness studies for all treatment methods. Require programs to report results, adverse effects, and morbidity and mortality of weight loss treatment. The weight loss industry needs to provide full disclosure and be held accountable for its results in the same way as other health care providers.

5. Knowledge

The needs for research and information in the weight and eating fields offer challenges in these areas:

■ Increase research of dysfunctional eating, eating disorders, size prejudice and overweight. More research, information and understanding is needed on causes, treatment and prevention; normal eating; body regulation of weight, hunger, appetite and satiety; physical and mental effects of starvation and semi-starvation; and the nature of the "thrifty gene" that impacts populations undergoing cultural change.

■ Encourage research and reporting in conferences and the scientific press by female researchers. Domination by males in research, publishing, scientific conferences, and health care policy has delayed recognition of the importance of women's issues in obesity and eating disorders, such as the role of sexual abuse in eating disorders.

■ Raise ethical standards. Loosen ties with weight loss industry at scientific conferences, on journal editorial boards and in public policy; require full disclosure of funding and business relationships. Obesity research has been particularly vulnerable to the power of vested interests, resulting in manipulation of data, evasion of the whole truth, and frequent reporting of short-term, irrelevant findings as if they were lasting and important.

■ Communicate research and information in effective ways to health care providers and consumers, keeping issues in perspective.

■ Consolidate eating and weight studies within one discipline, such as nutrition, while working closely with related fields, so the information can be researched, analyzed and used in a more comprehensive way than currently.

Appendix

Body Mass Index for Selected Weight and Stature

Stature m (in)

Weight kg (lb)	1.24 (49)	1.27 (50)	1.30 (51)	1.32 (52)	1.35 (53)	1.37 (54)	1.40 (55)	1.42 (56)	1.45 (57)	1.47 (58)	1.50 (59)	1.52 (60)	1.55 (61)	1.57 (62)	1.60 (63)	1.63 (64)	1.65 (65)	1.68 (66)	1.70 (67)	1.73 (68)	1.75 (69)	1.78 (70)	1.80 (71)	1.83 (72)	1.85 (73)	1.88 (74)	1.90 (75)	1.93 (76)
20 (45)	13	13	12	12	11	11	10	10	10	9	9	9	8															
23 (50)	15	14	13	13	12	12	12	11	11	10	10	10	9	9	9	9	8											
25 (55)	16	15	15	14	14	13	13	12	12	12	11	11	10	10	10	9	9	9										
27 (60)	18	17	16	16	15	15	14	13	13	13	12	12	11	11	11	10	10	10	9	9								
29 (65)	19	18	17	17	16	16	15	15	14	14	13	13	12	12	11	11	11	10	10	10								
32 (70)	21	20	19	18	17	17	16	16	15	15	14	14	13	13	12	12	12	11	11	11	10	10						
34 (75)	22	21	20	20	19	18	17	17	16	16	15	15	14	14	13	13	12	12	12	11	11	11	10					
36 (80)	24	22	21	21	20	19	19	18	17	17	16	16	15	15	14	14	13	13	13	12	12	11	11	11				
39 (85)	25	24	23	22	21	21	20	19	18	18	17	17	16	16	15	15	14	14	13	13	13	12	12	12				
41 (90)	27	25	24	23	22	22	21	20	19	19	18	18	17	17	16	15	15	14	14	14	13	13	13	12	12	12		
43 (95)	28	27	25	25	24	23	22	21	20	20	19	19	18	17	17	16	16	15	15	14	14	13	13	13	12	12		
45 (100)	29	28	27	26	25	24	23	22	22	21	20	20	19	18	18	17	17	16	16	15	15	14	14	14	13	13	13	12
48 (105)	31	30	28	27	26	25	24	24	23	22	21	21	20	19	19	18	17	17	16	16	15	15	14	14	13	13	13	
50 (110)	32	31	30	29	27	27	25	25	24	23	22	22	21	20	19	19	18	18	17	17	16	16	15	15	15	14	14	13
52 (115)	34	32	31	30	29	28	27	26	25	24	23	23	22	21	20	20	19	18	18	17	17	16	16	16	15	15	14	14
54 (120)	35	34	32	31	30	29	28	27	26	25	24	24	23	22	21	20	20	19	19	18	18	17	17	16	16	15	15	15
57 (125)	37	35	34	33	31	30	29	28	27	26	25	25	24	23	22	21	21	20	19	19	18	18	17	17	17	16	16	16
59 (130)	38	37	35	34	32	31	30	29	28	27	26	26	25	24	23	22	22	21	20	20	19	19	18	18	17	17	16	16
61 (135)	40	38	36	35	34	33	31	30	29	28	27	27	25	25	24	23	22	22	21	20	20	19	19	18	18	17	17	16
64 (140)	41	39	38	36	35	34	32	31	30	29	28	27	26	26	25	24	23	22	22	21	21	20	20	19	19	18	18	17
66 (145)	43	41	39	38	36	35	34	33	31	30	29	28	27	27	26	25	24	23	22	21	21	20	20	19	19	18	18	
68 (150)	44	42	40	39	37	36	35	34	32	31	30	29	28	28	27	26	25	24	24	23	22	21	21	20	20	19	19	18
70 (155)	46	44	42	40	39	37	36	35	33	33	31	30	29	29	27	26	26	25	24	23	23	22	22	21	21	20	19	19
73 (160)	47	45	43	42	40	39	37	36	35	34	32	31	30	29	28	27	27	26	25	24	23	22	22	21	21	20	20	19
77 (170)	50	48	46	44	42	41	39	38	37	36	34	33	32	31	30	29	28	27	27	26	25	24	24	23	23	22	21	21
79 (175)		49	47	46	44	42	40	39	38	37	35	34	33	32	31	30	29	28	27	27	26	25	24	24	23	22	22	21
82 (180)		51	48	47	45	44	42	40	39	38	36	35	34	33	32	31	30	29	28	27	27	26	25	24	24	23	23	22
84 (185)		50	48	47	45	44	42	41	40	38	37	36	35	34	33	32	31	30	29	28	27	27	26	25	25	24	23	23
86 (190)				49	47	46	44	43	41	40	39	37	36	35	34	32	32	31	30	29	28	27	27	26	25	24	24	23
88 (195)				51	49	47	45	44	42	41	39	38	37	36	35	33	32	31	31	30	29	28	27	26	26	25	25	24
91 (200)					50	48	46	45	43	42	40	40	38	37	35	34	33	32	31	30	29	28	27	27	26	25	25	24
93 (205)							50	47	46	44	43	41	40	39	38	36	35	34	33	32	31	30	29	28	27	26	26	25
95 (210)							49	47	45	44	42	41	40	39	37	36	35	34	33	32	31	30	29	28	28	27	26	26
98 (215)							50	48	46	45	43	42	41	40	38	37	36	35	34	33	32	31	30	29	28	28	27	26
100 (220)								49	47	46	44	43	42	40	39	38	37	35	35	33	33	31	31	30	30	29	28	27
102 (225)								51	49	47	45	44	42	41	40	38	37	36	35	34	33	32	31	30	30	29	28	27
104 (230)									50	48	46	45	43	42	41	39	38	37	36	35	34	33	32	31	30	30	29	28
107 (235)										49	47	46	44	43	42	40	39	38	37	36	35	34	33	32	31	30	30	29
109 (240)										50	48	47	45	44	43	41	40	39	38	36	36	34	34	33	32	31	31	30
111 (245)										49	48	46	45	43	42	41	40	39	38	37	36	35	34	33	32	31	31	30
113 (250)											50	49	47	46	44	43	42	40	39	38	37	36	35	34	33	32	31	30
116 (255)												50	48	47	45	44	42	41	40	39	38	37	36	35	34	33	32	31
118 (260)												49	48	46	44	43	42	41	39	39	38	37	36	35	34	33	33	32
120 (265)													50	49	47	45	44	43	42	40	39	38	37	36	35	34	33	32
122 (270)														50	48	46	45	43	42	41	40	39	38	37	36	35	34	33
125 (275)														49	47	46	44	43	42	41	39	38	38	37	36	35	35	33
127 (280)															50	48	47	45	44	42	41	40	39	38	37	36	35	34
129 (285)															50	49	47	46	45	43	42	41	40	39	38	37	36	35
132 (290)																50	48	47	46	44	43	42	41	39	38	37	36	35
134 (295)																50	49	47	46	45	44	42	41	40	39	38	37	36
136 (300)																	50	48	47	45	44	43	42	41	40	39	38	37

GAPS: Adolescent Preventive Services
American Medical Association

The American Medical Association recognizes the crisis in adolescent health and recommends a fundamental change aimed at prevention. AMA's new GAPS program (Guidelines for Adolescent Preventive Services) calls for health care providers to screen teenagers each year on weight and eating issues, along with other major health risks. Following is information from the 1995 GAPS Recommendations Monograph on how to deal with the current health crisis for adolescents:

"Changes in adolescent morbidity and mortality during the past several decades have created a health crisis for today's youth. Unintended pregnancy, STDs including HIV, alcohol and drug abuse, and eating disorders are just some of the health problems faced by an increasing number of adolescents from all sectors of society.

"This health crisis requires a fundamental change in the emphasis of adolescent services — a change whereby a greater number of services are directed at the primary and secondary prevention of the major health threats facing today's youth. School and community organizations have responded to the need for change by increasing health education programming. Primary care physicians and other health providers must respond by making preventive services a greater component of their clinical practice."

GAPS recommends preventive screening and health promotion for eating disorders and obesity during annual health visits between age 11 and 21,

- All adolescents should be screened annually for eating disorders and obesity by determining weight and stature, and asking about body image and dieting patterns.

- Adolescents should be assessed for organic disease, anorexia nervosa, or bulimia if any of the following are found: weight loss greater than 10% of previous weight; recurrent dieting when not overweight; use of self-induced emesis, laxatives, starvation, or diuretics to lose weight; distorted body image; or body mass index (BMI) below the 5th percentile.

■ Adolescents with a BMI equal to or greater than the 95th percentile for age and gender are overweight and should have an in-depth dietary and health assessment to determine psychosocial morbidity and risk for future cardiovascular disease.

■ Adolescents with a BMI between the 85th and 94th percentile are at risk for becoming overweight. A dietary and health assessment to determine psychosocial morbidity and risk for future cardiovascular disease should be performed on these youth if:

- their BMI has increased by two or more units during the previous 12 months;

- there is a family history of premature heart disease, obesity, hypertension, or diabetes mellitus;

- they express concern about their weight;

- they have elevated serum cholesterol levels or blood pressure.

■ If this assessment is negative, these adolescents should be provided general dietary and exercise counseling and should be monitored annually.

AMA calls the GAPS recommendations a major change from the traditional approach to adolescent health care, which focused on and treated specific biomedical problems alone. In the new approach the health provider plays an important role in coordinating adolescent health promotion by complementing the guidance received from family, school and community, whereas in the past it was considered to be independent.

GAPS emphasizes screening for comorbidities and early detection of health problems through the annual visits. These visits offer an opportunity to provide health education and develop a therapeutic relationship. The provider performs three comprehensive physical examinations: one during early, middle and late adolescence.

It is recommended that all parents receive education about adolescent health care at least twice during their child's adolescence.

The emphasis is on comprehensive assessment and early detection of health problems.

The AMA offers a training program for physicians on how to

deliver these kinds of clinical preventive services and help patients change behavior. This first step by AMA will be followed by more specific recommendations on prevention and treatment.

AMA resources for adolescent health care and screening include:
AMA Guidelines for Adolescent Preventive Services:
Recommendations and Rationale
Clinical Evaluation and Management Handbook
Implementation and Resource Manual
Implementation Training Workshop
GAPS Presentation Kit
Implementation Forms
Culturally Competent Health Care for Adolescents
Also: Policy recommendations on critical health issues of adolescents, made by major medical and allied health associations for: tobacco, alcohol, other harmful substances, violence, intentional injury, abuse, reproductive health issues affecting adolescents.

Information and materials available from:
Department of Adolescent Health
American Medical Association
515 North State Street
Chicago, IL 60610
(312-464-5570; fax 312-464-5842)

Complications of Eating Disorders

Mental complications

Anorexia Nervosa

Many of the mental and emotional symptoms common to anorexia nervosa are directly related to the physical effects of starvation. These are documented in wartime Keys Minnesota Starvation Study in which 32 men underwent dramatic personality changes during six months on half rations, when they lost one-fourth of their weight. Other traits have to do with attitudes and behavior toward eating and weight. The following are psychological traits commonly associated with anorexia nervosa.10

- Energy level. Fatigue, weakness, lassitude, lethargy, apathy, decreasing energy, persistent tiredness dizziness, faintness, light-headedness, yet compulsively exercises (hyperactive).

- Mood, attitude and behavior. Moodiness, often depressed or irritable, mood swings (tyrannical); anxiety and ambivalence; irritability; critical; less tolerant of others; depression; low self-esteem, self-esteem control through weight loss; invulnerability and success dependent on weight loss; feelings of lack of control in life; hopelessness; rigidity, highly controlled behavior; does not reveal feelings; perfectionist behavior; fantasy that weight loss can cause or prevent some life event (prevent parental divorce, attract romance); denies hunger; denies problem of weight loss (sees self as fat); denies eating disorder; body image distortion (overestimates body size and shape, "feels fat" despite emaciated appearance); ritualistic habits.

- Mental ability. Inability to concentrate, decreased alertness; difficulty with reading comprehension, diminished capacity to think; loss of memory; extreme narrowing of interests; decline in ambition.

- Social. Social withdrawal, isolates self from family and friends, becomes increasingly aloof and withdrawn; loneliness; feelings easily hurt; avoidance by peers; worsening family relations, fights with family, cost of treatment may be financial drain.

- Weight. increasing preoccupation with body; frequently monitors body changes (may check with scale and/or mirror many times per day); compares size and shape to others, envious of thinner persons; heightened control, feelings of having control over body.

- Food, eating and hunger. Misperception of hunger, satiety and other bodily sensations; hunger and increasing hunger; fears food and gaining weight; eats alone; guilt when eating; may secretly binge; dieting and weight increasingly important focus; unusual food-related behaviors (makes rules for specific foods, placement on plate, time of eating, size of bites, number of chews per bite); progressive preoccupation with food and eating (may begin to cook and control family's eating); need to vicariously enjoy food (may collect recipes, dream of food, hoard food, enjoy watching others eat, pursue food-related careers — as dietitians, chefs, caterers).

- Other. Hypersensitive to cold and heat, hypersensitive to noise and light; sleep disturbance.

Bulimia nervosa

When a patient with anorexia becomes bulimic, she or he experiences symptoms characteristic of both eating disorders. The woman with bulimia nervosa is often normal weight and may not experience the effects of starvation. However, if she has severe nutrition deficiencies due to purging, she may have some of the same starvation symptoms.

Typically, these mental and emotional symptoms may be associated with bulimia nervosa:

- Mood/attitude/behavior. Anxiety, depression; mood swings; low self-esteem, self-deprecating thoughts; embarrassment, shame related to behavior; persistent remorse; paranoid feelings; unreasonable resentments; makes excuses to go to restroom after meals; may buy large amounts of food, which suddenly disappears, impulsive as compared to anorexics who are overcontrolled.

- Mental ability. Loss of ordinary willpower, poor impulse control, self-indulgent behavior; recognizes abnormal eating behavior.

- Social. Depends on others for approval; feelings of isolation; unable to discuss problem, others unhappy about food obsession; social isolation; distances self from friends and family; fear of going out in public; family, work and money problems.

- Weight. Feels that self worth is dependent on low weight; constant concern with weight and body image.

- Food, eating and hunger. Eats alone; eats when not hungry; preoccupation with eating and food; fears binges and eating out of control; increased dependency on bingeing; binge eating of large amount of food in a short time, feeling out of control, cannot stop eating.

- Purging. Feels need to rid body of calories consumed during binge (through vomiting, laxatives, diuretics, enemas, fasting or excessive exercise); experimentation with vomiting, laxatives and diuretics often leads to regular abuse.

- Binge/purge cycle. Spends much time planning, carrying out, cleaning up after bulimic episode; eliminates normal activities; complex lifestyle may develop with episodes occurring several times a day; worsening of symptoms during times of emotional stress; feels soothed and comforted by binge/purge cycle — it may serve to relieve frustration, anxiety, anger, fear, remorse, boredom, loneliness.

■ Other. Dishonesty, lying; stealing food or money; drug and alcohol abuse; suicidal tendencies or attempts.

Physical complications

Anorexia Nervosa

■ Electrolytes. May be low in potassium, sodium, chloride, calcium, magnesium, and high or low bicarbonate. Electrolyte imbalance more likely when there is dehydration and/or purging.

■ Gastrointestinal. Constipation is likely, may promote laxative use. Commonly there is vomiting, feelings of fullness and bloating, and abdominal discomfort. There may be ulcers, and pancreatic dysfunction. Excessive laxatives over time may result in gastrointestinal bleeding and impairment of colon functioning.

■ Cardiovascular. Commonly present are chest pain, arrhythmias, hypotension, edema and mitral valve prolapse. Electrocardiogram (EKG) changes. Heart rates lower than 40 beats per minute are common and as low as 25 reported in severe starvation. Prolonged QT intervals can lead to sudden death syndrome.

■ Metabolic. Abnormal temperature regulation and cold intolerance are common. Abnormal glucose tolerance, fasting hypoglycemia, high B-hydroxybutyric acid, high free fatty acids, hypercholesterolemia, hypercarotenemia are common. Diabetic patients with an eating disorder may have fluctuating blood glucose levels leading to serious longterm consequences.

■ Bones. Decreased bone mineral density may lead to fractures, growth retardation, short stature and osteoporosis.

■ Renal. Elevated blood urea nitrogen, changes in urinary concentration capacity, and decreased glomerular filtration rate are common.

■ Endocrine. Amenorrhea is 100%, by definition, although many anorexia nervosa patients begin to menstruate over time. Related to weight loss but may precede weight loss (in one-third); may cause delayed puberty, contributes to osteoporosis, breast atrophy, infertility. Hypometabolic state resulting in cold intolerance, dry skin and hair, bradycardia, constipation, fatigue, slowed reflexes. High plasma cortisol, decreased cortixol response to insulin.

■ Hematologic. Anemia, leukopenia, bone marrow hypocellularity, common; these effects are usually mild, but can include bleeding tendency.

- Neurological. EEG and sleep changes are common; epileptic seizures affect up to 10 percent.
- Musculocutaneous. Muscle weakening, muscle cramps. Hair loss, brittle hair and nails, lanugo hair, dry skin and cold extremities are common.

Bulimia nervosa

- Electrolytes. Low potassium, low chloride, dehydration and metabolic alkalosis are common. May lead to cardiac arrest, renal failure. Dehydration is common along with hypotension, dizziness, weakness, muscle cramps. Cardiac arrhythmias affect 20 percent; unpredictable, may require emergency treatment.

  Hypochloremia is common; limits kidney's ability to excrete bicarbonate.

- Gastrointestinal. Constipation and increased amylase common. Rarely gastric and duodenal ulcer, acute gastric dilation and rupture. Frequent abdominal pain. Severe abdominal pain may lead to rigid abdomen and shock which may result in death. Abuses of laxatives may lead to iron deficiency anemia, rectal bleeding and cathartic colon.
- Pulmonary. Aspiration pneumonia possible from aspiration of vomitus.
- Cardiovascular. Peripheral edema is common along with EKG changes and QT changes, which can lead to serious arrhythmias and congestive heart failure. Uncommon is sudden cardiac death. Ipecac syrup abuse may lead to death through cardiomyopathy, myocarditis.
- Metabolic. High B-hydroxybutyric acid, free fatty acids. Less common edema, abnormal temperature regulation and cold intolerance.
- Renal. Possible changes.
- Endocrine. Menstrual irregularities with low body weight, dexamethasone nonsuppression common.
- Hematologic. May be anemic with nutrition deficiency.
- Neurological. EEG changes common. May have epileptic seizures with malnutrition and electrolyte imbalance.
- Musculocutaneous. Calluses on dorsum of dominant hand are common from inducing gag reflex. Muscle weakening with ipecac abuse.
- Dental. Enamel erosions with vomiting.

Compiled from: Kaplan A, and P Garfinkel, Medical issues and the Eating Disorders, 1993, Brunner/Mazel, New York, NY.

Dysfunctional eating
Research basis

Among the important sources on which the concept of dysfunctional eating is built are: the early work on restrained eating by Janet Polivy and Peter Herman[1]; writings and presentations by Susan Wooley[2]; writings and work by Ellyn Satter on normal eating and her workshops on "Treating the dieting casualty"[3]; Linda Omichinski's nondiet leadership and program development devoted to breaking the dieting cycle[4]; the concept development on thinking about food by Dan and Kim Reiff;[5] starvation studies, including the Minnesota Experiment[6] United Nations reports on world malnutrition[7], and Colin Turnbull's striking portrait of *The Mountain People*[8]; national and local studies showing the high prevalence of dieting and disordered eating among children and adolescents[9]; eating disorder research showing mental and physical effects of eating disorders, and the associations of eating disorders with dieting[10]; discussions on the risks of dieting and the need to treat chronic dieting syndrome by Arnold Andersen and Mike Bowers[11]; and the evolution of No Diet Day developments, led by Mary Evans Young,[12] and Eating Disorder Awareness Week, led by eating disorder specialists.[13]

Most of this information has been reviewed in *Healthy Weight Journal* over the past 11 years, and is discussed extensively and referenced in the book *Health Risks of Weight Loss.*[14]

References
1. Herman P, J Polivy. Eating and its disorders, edit Stunkard and Steller, 1984, 141-56. Raven Press.
   Healthy Weight J Mar/Apr 1996;10:2:32-33.
2. Wooley S, W Wooley. Eating and its disorders, edit Stunkard and Steller, 1984. Raven Press.
3. Satter, Ellyn, How to get your kids to eat — but not too much, Bull PUbl, Palo Alto, CA.
   Workshops, "Treating the dieting casualty," Satter Assoc., Madison, WI.
4. Omichinski L, You Count, Calories Don't, 1992; HUGS facilitator programs, HUGS International, Box 102A, Rt3, Portage la Prairie, Manitoba, R1N 3A3, Canada; Teens & Diets — No Weigh, Healthy Weight J 1996;10:3:49-52; Berg F, Nondiet movement gains strength

HWJ/Obesity & Health Sep/Oct 1992;6:5:82-90.

5. Reiff D, KK Lampson Reiff, Eating Disorders: Nutrition Therapy in the Recovery Process, 1992. Aspen, Gaithersburg, MD; Personal communication with Dan Reiff, 1996.

6. Keys A, et al. Biology of human starvation, 1950. U of Minn Press, Minneapolis, MN.

    Berg F, Starvation stages in weight loss patients similar to famine victims, HWJ/Obesity & Health Apr 1989;3:4:27-30.

7. Body Mass Index. FAO, A measure of chronic energy deficiency in adults, 1994, United Nations report.

    Berg F, World starvation: weight may be best tool to measure malnutrition, Healthy Weight J May/Jun 1995;9:3:47-49.

8. Turnbull, Colin, 1972, The Mountain People. Simon and Schuster, NY.

9. CDC USHHS, Behavioral Risk Survey; Calorie Control Council, 1991 National Survey.

    Berg F, Who is dieting in the U.S. Healthy Weight Journal/Obesity & Health 1992;6:3:48-49.

    Dieting and purging behavior in black and white high school students, JADA 1992;92:3:306-312.

    Adolescents dieting; JAMA 1991;266:2811-2812.

    Berg F, Harmful weight loss practices among adolescents, HWJ/ O&H Jul/Aug 1992;6:4:69-72.

10. Fallon P, Katzman M, Wooley S, Feminist perspectives on eating disorders 1994, Guilford Press, NY.

    Baker D, R Sansone, Overview of eating disorders, 1994:1-10, NEDO.

    Kaplan A, P Garfinkel, Medical issues and the eating disorders, 1993, Brunner/Mazel, NY.

    Berg F, Eating disorders: physical and mental effects, Healthy Weight J Mar/Apr 1995;9:2:27-30.

    Smolak L, M Levine, Toward an empirical basis for primary prevention of eating problems with elementary school children, Eat Disorders 1994;2:4:293-307

11. Andersen A. The last word, Eating Disorders 1994;2:1:81-82.

    Bowers M. The last word. Eating Disorders 1994;2:4:375-377.

12. Young, Mary Evans, Diet Breaking, 1996, Hodder & Stoughton, London.

13. Biely J, Eating Disorder Awareness Week '96, EDAP Matters Winter 1996;2.

14. Berg F. Health Risks of Weight Loss, 1995. Chapter 1. General treatment risks, 14-26; Ch 7. Eating disorders, 56-62; Ch 8. Psychological risks, 63-69; Ch 9. Weight cycling, 70-79; Ch 11. Thinness: a cultural obsession, 89-99; Ch 13. To treat or not to treat, 108-113. 66:2811-2812; Berg F, Harmful weight loss practices among adolescents, HWJ/O&H Jul/Aug 1992;6:4:69.

Radical animal rights agenda

"A rat is a pig is a dog is a boy."

Seattle Times, 9-11-89: The dangerous campaign being waged by the animal-rights activists is not a struggle against medical science alone; it is a struggle against humanity.

American Medical Association: A humane concern for the welfare of animals means wanting to see that they are treated without cruelty, are properly cared for and not made to suffer unnecessary pain. That's right and good. But that is quite unlike the fanaticism of the animal rights extremists. Some of these extremists . . . have vandalized labs, set them on fire, destroyed research files, harassed scientists and technicians, and issued death threats.

Alex Pacheco, one of PETA's founders, has said that, "Arson, property destruction, burglary or theft are acceptable crimes when they directly alleviate the pain and suffering of an animal."

Ingrid Newkirk heads People for the Ethical Treatment of Animals, or PETA . . . one of perhaps more than 400 such animal rights organizations across the country. She once said on a radio talk show that morally there is no basic difference between human beings and other animals, "A rat is a pig is a dog is a boy."

American Medical Association presentation: It seems to me you can't argue that human beings are morally the same as animals, and then also argue that we should behave differently toward animals than they behave toward each other — or us, given the chance.

Nature is beautiful, but it is also harsh. To survive, most organisms eat other organisms, either plant or animal. And there are many places in the world where careless humans still become dinner for tigers, sharks, crocodiles, piranha and other predators. I doubt if they worry much about the morality of eating a human being.

The fact is, we are the only species that does worry about these things. Besides our complex languages, our free will and our reason, we are the only animals with a moral sensibility — and that does set us apart. In fact, that's why we care about the humane treatment of animals . . . (but) polls show that the American public overwhelmingly rejects the activists' claim that there is no difference between animals and humans.

The Gallup Youth Survey: We are an animal loving nation, and so it should come as no surprise that as children who have been devoted to their dogs,

What do animal rights activists want?

Agenda of the animal "rights" movement:
- Elimination of animals in research
- No meat, dairy products
- No leather, silk
- No zoos, circuses, aquariums
- No pets

Tactics of some animal "rights" groups:
- Public disinformation campaign
- Arson
- Destruction of medical research laboratories, offices, files
- Bombings
- Harassment
- Death threats

Animal "rights": Abolish use of animals for food, clothes, pets, medical education and research

By contrast, animal welfare concerns: Responsible care, preventing cruelty, support for neutering and adoption

AMERICAN MEDICAL ASSOCIATION

cats and hamsters grow older, they become highly supportive of efforts to protect animal species that are endangered.

The scientific and medical communities probably will be alarmed, however, to discover that according to the findings of the most recent Gallup Youth Survey, a majority of the nation's teenagers also say they support the "animal rights movement," even if it would mean the end to laboratory and medical tests that use animals . . .

A plurality of 41 percent support the movement very much, and are joined by 26 percent who say they are somewhat in favor of it. Among the remaining teens, 18 percent say they are somewhat opposed to animal rights, 14 percent are very much opposed, and 3 percent have no opinion about the movement . . . As teens grow older their support diminishes somewhat.

— George Gallup, Jr., and Alec Gallup, 1991

Wall street Journal 9-2-92: Major groups such as PETA have found big success in attracting young members, after-school animal-rights clubs have sprung up across the country, and the Dissection Hotline set up to counsel students has received 40,000 calls in three years, says its director, Pat Graham.

Part of the reason for the youth explosion is PETA's success at making animal rights a hip cause. In addition to school mailings, teens have flocked to the movement after seeing endorsements by movie stars. PETA also sets up tables at concerts by such groups as Guns N' Roses.

High schoolers aren't the only new advocates, either. Nearly 5,000 subscribers under age 10 receive a magazine called PETA Kids, featuring cartoons and connect-the-dots puzzles, along with advice on how to become a vegetarian and how to prevent animal cruelty.

American Medical Association statement: Virtually all medical advances in the 20th century have required laboratory animal research, including vaccines for polio and measles, cancer chemotherapy, open heart surgery, and insulin for diabetics.

Nancy Tullis, RD, Reliable Nutrition Information Chair of the Louisville Dietetic Association, Louisville, Ky: Farmers could not stay in business by treating animals inhumanely — they would not grow properly or would die of sickness. Why not attack a perceived problem directly by reporting to authorities, instead of by the passive self-denial of not eating veal? The gross treatment of animals as shown on the EarthSave video in schools is emotional blackmail.

Self appointed "nutritionists" should not be allowed to go into the schools to present an emotional diatribe about society's shortcomings in the areas of nutrition, air, soil, water and animal cruelty, place blame on certain groups, and then irresponsibly teach the new vegan diet pattern, leaving some inadequate brochures behind. The children will go home short on facts and long on anger. We do not believe in setting children up for this emotional confrontation with their families.

Edwin Locke, PhD, College of Business and Management, University of Maryland, College Park: Animal rights advocates (at least the leaders) are the ones who are anti-life; their hatred of man is openly and loudly proclaimed. They must be fought and stopped in the name of morality.

World Medical Association Statement, France, 1989: Biomedical research is essential to the health and well-being of every person in our society.

Advances have dramatically improved the quality and prolonged the duration of life throughout the world.

However, the ability of the scientific community to continue its efforts to improve personal and public health is being threatened by a movement to eliminate the use of animals. This movement is spearheaded by groups of radical animal rights activists whose views are far outside mainstream public attitudes and whose tactics range from sophisticated lobbying, fund raising, propaganda and misinformation campaigns to violent attacks on research facilities and individual scientists.

The magnitude of violent animal rights activities is staggering. In the U.S. alone, since 1980, animal rights groups have staged more than 29 raids on U.S. research facilities, stealing over 2,000 animals, causing more than 7 million dollars in physical damages and ruining years of scientific research. Animal activist groups have engaged in similar activities in Great Britain, Western Europe, Canada and Australia. Various groups in these countries have claimed responsibility for the bombing of cars, institutions, stores, and the private homes of researchers.

Constance Horner, U.S. Under Secretary of Health and Human Services, 1990: Ingrid Newkirk has equated the death of chickens with the deaths of people who died in concentration camps during World War II. The idea of animal rights may set out to insure that animals are treated as human beings, but by blurring the essential distinction between the two, it lends itself just as readily to the suggestion that human beings may be treated as animals. And given the history of the twentieth century and the sufferings of millions around the world, there is clear danger that the latter interpretation will enjoy ascendancy.

Thus the doctrine that purports to elevate the status of all living things is, in the end, a doctrine that debases the status of mankind, and endangers our essential freedoms.

Jon Franklin, Professor of Journalism, University of Oregon, Eugene: That's what they are saying now — "Let the crippled children die." You think not? You think they haven't gone that far? Well, read Peter Singer's latest book, "Should the Baby Live? The Problem of Handicapped Infants." He's the Australian philosopher who wrote "Animal Liberation."

These folks routinely compare scientists to Nazis . . . Yet Hitler, too . . . thought it better to experiment on humans . . . like the animal rights advocates . . . There are similarities . . . The attitude toward crippled children, for instance, and the ethics of human experimentation. In the first place, Adolf Hitler himself was an animal "rights" person and a vegetarian. This is a fact. Goebels, who was proud of shunning the small lie, promised on a variety of public occasions that one feature of the Third Reich would be a new respect for animals, and a phasing out of animal experimentation.

At the same time the Nazi party was busy anthropomorphizing animals it was also at work dehumanizing not just the Jews but generally people who were not up to what was considered par, physically and mentally. Listen closely to the words of animal rights advocates. Do you detect the dehumanizition of certain groups?

Michael Kerr, The Seattle Times, 5-1-91: The other day I attended a religious revival . . . the local meeting of the Progressive Animal Welfare Society (PAWS). Members of the latest, fastest-growing, and most politically correct religion on the block — the religion of animal rights. I knew that animal-rights activists existed, but I never thought they were important — just some people who, if ignored long enough, would fade away. Attendance at a single PAWS meeting proved me wrong.

I sat through the meeting in a state of shock. The information fed to the audience was so exaggerated, misinformed, inflammatory, and sometimes so wrong that I kept wondering if it were some kind of joke — but the people in the audience believed every word.

They are in a holy mission of intimidation and misinformation to spread the Truth. And, in the environmentally sensitive culture we have now, the message is spreading.

Animal rights are becoming the "hot new issue of the '90s". . . (But) the money you send for PAWS' low-cost neutering clinics might be used to shut down a research laboratory that could find a cure for AIDS. The money you send to stop fur trapping might be used in the campaign against research in brain injuries.

NOTE TO THE MEDIA: Writers, editors and producers need to be aware of their potential manipulation by animal rights activists and the "political correctness" the media has already accorded them. For example, the press recently attacked a young boy with an incurable illness who asked, for his Make-a-Wish desire, for the opportunity to hunt big game in Alaska. Instead of destroying the dreams of a young boy, the press would better have investigated and reported on the source of these attacks. At the very least, it can ignore them. Loving and caring for animals is very different from the chilling radical animal rights agenda.

The American Medical Association maintains a press office at its headquarters in Chicago that will answer media questions on animal rights issues.

Working with teenagers

Teens & Diets: No Weigh

How to deliver the nondieting message

by Linda Omichinski, RD

The importance of breaking the diet cycle at an early age can't be overemphasized. As health professionals we can take some new directions and responsibility to change the cultural message.

What legacy are we passing on to the next generation? Are we a society of dieters unhappy with the way we look because media messages tell us we should be slim? Food preoccupation and dieting has become an obsession for too many. The right to enjoy food and accept the inherent satisfaction and sustainment that comes from nourishing your body seems to have been stolen away.

The good news is that healthy, nondieting is a valid lifestyle choice that comes with a freeing set of parameters and characteristics far surpassing the restrictions of a diet lifestyle. There is no better time for establishing a new way of living than the teen years.

Working with teens

We decided to get involved with nondiet programming for teens because of several compelling factors.

From our facilitator network we were hearing comments like . . . "There's nothing out there for teens that isn't weight loss," " I'm counseling too many kids with eating disorders," "Parents in my group said they'd like this for their teen."

Diet myths and diet mentality are entrenched in our culture. Curriculum and programs in schools are loaded with diet and weight bias. Educators are inadvertently passing on myths, fallacies and mixed messages simply because alternate material hasn't existed.

Part of working with teens involves letting go of the control and enabling them to make the decisions. Comments like, "That's a very interesting point of view. Could you tell me more about that?" lets the teen express their own perspective.

Empowerment techniques are ideally suited for teen development.

It's critical to have an open attitude about the seeming negatives in this age group so that true learning can take place. Personal qualities of openness, caring and a good sense of humor aid educators of any age group and particularly for teens.

Build a relationship based on trust; share personal stories and some background so they can identify with you. Treat teens as adults, with the acceptance that will enable feeling good, relaxing and opening up to occur. Emphasize that no question is stupid. Use lots of humor.

Be watchful for fear in the group and offer reassurance and support for the courage to try something new. Build flexibility within the structure of your time together and introduce new concepts very gradually. Take the time to appreciate where they are in their maturity and background as a group and individually. Understand the range of behaviors and accept that everyone learns a different way. It often takes time for teens to buy into the dynamics of a group. Not everyone is ready for the same message at the same time or able to implement the ideas in their own situation — we all grow at a different pace.

When you are in a leadership role, the words you use, particularly in a one-on-one situation, can have permanent impact. The message received may not always be the one you intended to deliver. And, it's not just the words, but the tone that delivers the message. Your aim is to nurture, assist and guide; not destroy and break down.

Encourage feedback from others to see if your verbal reflection matches your intent. Find out what words will encourage and empower teens to become stronger, healthier people. Words can be verbal shoves, especially to those with undeveloped or low self-esteem. With teens the unexpected should be expected so that your non-judgmental tones have to be always ready. An attitude of casual but respectful curiosity encourages frankness.

What schools are teaching

We recommend four prongs to reach the public with a nondieting health message for teens: through schools, teen grapevines, parental concern, and the medical/health professional community

We identified six areas of concern with schools:

1. "Correct weight" references and material. Measures and figures such as BMI (body mass index) and height/weight charts, weigh-ins, and use of skin calipers carry the potential to seriously affect self-esteem.
2. Focus on weight instead of health. Students need to feel an appreciation of different body shapes and sizes. Weight is determined by one's genetic predisposition, history of chronic dieting and lifestyle.
3. Showing students how to lose weight instead of emphasizing the living concepts (eat and exercise for energy and fun), and accept the weight that grows out of that. Otherwise, perfectionist tendencies, and preoccupation with weight can arise.

Teens & Diets - No Weigh

Program goals

- Establish a lifestyle perspective for young people to take responsibility for their own food needs   and activities.
- Enable teens to take responsibility for their own eating preferences.
- Help teens understand and incorporate into their own lives the interconnectedness of food, activity and attitude.
- Provide knowledge, instill skills and build confidence so that young people are equipped to find their personal balance of food and physical activity to energize their lifestyle choices.
- Involve the family unit in the process of understanding the necessity for individual patterns of nourishment.
- Provide information about body image and self-esteem.
- Provide new knowledge about food.
- Provide new knowledge about physical activity.
- Demonstrate how to be experimental and assertive.

For the teen

- How to take responsibility for own appetite and tastes within the family setting.
- How to understand signals in own body for hunger.
- How to use consistent physical activity as a source of energy.
- How to eat for energy and health.
- How to appreciate genetic and growth factors in personal appearance changes.
- How to have a healthier body image.
- How to express oneself assertively.
- How to critically look at media messages around health/body image.
- How to measure health as a state of energetic and confident well-being as opposed to a number on the scale.

For the family

- Respect individual food preferences.
- Offer a variety of foods.
- Understand physical differences in the need for food.
- Convey non-judgmental attitudes.
- Demonstrate unreserved acceptance of teen.

From the HUGS for Teens program, Teens & Diets - No Weigh: Building the road to healthier living, 1995, by Linda Omichinski, RD.

CHILDREN AND TEENS IN WEIGHT CRISIS 1995

4. The Food Pyramid contains useful information about the roles of foods. But good food/bad food connotations often arise during discussions that stick with people's permanent perception of the food.
5. A widespread "fat is bad" bandwagon. Fats are essential for a healthy body as they supply energy (fat soluble vitamins and fatty acids) and/or other important nutrients to help teens grow.
6. Often one or two competitive sports dominate the focus of acceptable physical activity. The public school system can and should provide opportunities to experiment with different types of activities. Teens should be able to experience a range of activities to discover ones that are personally enjoyable.

One parent summarized thoughtfully . . . "The idea of not having to diet made them relax and not be so anxious about eating (as that made them eat more), also the knowledge of their different food choices and the help with making the right choices was good. This program was helpful, as they get tired of their mother telling them, they can just refer back to the info they received from this program."

Another mother felt her daughter really benefited from the program as she now eats breakfast.

One program facilitator delivered classes through a community health service because the content met the criteria of the region's business plan to empower people to be the best they can be. A strength is that the material on teen smoking fits the goal of decreasing the incidence of smoking. The program was delivered at the junior high school and will later be brought into the senior high school level.

Another said, "The concept of the program is terrific. It is just the thing that most teens need. So many teens go on diets — more so than adults — creating a great need for this program. Hopefully, we will be able to reach a lot of teens and show them that diets don't work. Overall, the program was a success. Most of the teens really enjoyed the program."

Registered dietitian and nondiet leader Linda Omichinski provides readers with a look inside her new program Teens & Diets: No Weigh.

Reprinted with permission from the HUGS teen facilitator package Teens & Diets: No Weigh, by Linda Omichinski, Copyright 1995. HUGS International Inc., Box 102A, RR#3, Portage la Prairie, Manitoba, R1N 3A3, Canada (1-800-565-4847).

Child-centered resources
The health promotion approach

Kid's Project, Packet of size acceptance materials from the Council on Size & Weight Discrimination, Miriam Berg, P.O. Box 305, Mt. Marion, NY 12456 (914-679-1209; fax 914-679-1206).

Good News for Big Kids. National Association to Advance Fat Acceptance. Pamphlet. NAAFA, PO Box 188620, Sacramento, CA 95818 (1-800-442-1214; 916-558-6880; fax 916-558-6881).

Am I Fat? Helping Young Children Accept Differences in Body Size, by Joanne Ikeda, MA, RD, and Priscilla Naworski, MS, CHES. Softcover, 110 pages. ETR Associates, PO Box 1830, Santa Cruz, CA 95061-1880 (1-800-321-4407).

If My Child is Too Fat, What should I do about it? Booklet for parents by Joanne Ikeda (501-642-2790; fax 510-642-0535).
Children and Weight: What's a parent to do? and **Family Choices for Good Health**. Low-literacy booklets for parents by Joanne Ikeda and Rita Mitchell. ANR Publications, University of California, 6701 San Pablo Ave., Oakland, CA 94608 (415-642-2431).

Children and Weight: What's a parent to do? 12-minute videotape, includes sample parent books. English and Spanish. Visual Media, 1441 Research Park Drive, University of California, Davis, CA 95616.

How to get your Kid to Eat — But not too much, by Ellyn Satter. Birth through adolescence, 1987, softcover, 396 pages. Bull Publishing.
Child of Mine — Feeding with love and good sense, by Ellyn Satter. Pregnancy through toddler stage, 1983, softcover. Bull Publishing,, Box 208, Palo Alto, CA 94302 (415-322-2855).

Feeding with Love and Good Sense, by Ellyn Satter. Series of four 15-minute videotapes about the feeding relationship for the infant, older baby, toddler and the preschooler, set of four on one tape. Ellyn Satter Associates.
Feeding with Love and Good Sense Training Manual, 103 pages, includes rights to reproduce teaching materials. **Ellyn Satter's Vision workshop**. Ellen Satter Assoc., 4226 Mandan Crescent, Madison, WI 53711 (1-800-808-7976; fax 608-271-7976).

Teens & Diets — No Weigh: Building the road to healthier living. A HUGS for Teens program franchised to licensed health professionals, by Linda Omichinski, RD. Eight lesson plans, scripts and resources. Supported with Tailoring Your Tastes, teen journal, parent guide handbook, 1995. HUGS International, Box 102A, RR3, Portage la Prairie, Manitoba, Canada R1N 3A3 (204-428-3432; 1-800-565-4847; fax 204-428-5072).

Vitality Leader's Kit. Contains Vitality health promotion materials that focus on a fundamental shift from treatment to prevention of weight problems including overweight, underweight, eating disorders, weight preoccupation and negative body image, 1994. Health Services and Promotion, Health and Welfare Canada, 4th Floor, Jeanne Mance Bldg., Ottawa, Ontario, Canada K1A 1B4 (613-957-8331; fax 613-941-2399).

References

Chapter 1
1. P.L.E.A.S.E. Newsl. Spring-Summer 1996;2.
2. Natl Ctr for Health Statistics, NHANES III. Advance Data Nov 14, 1994.
3. Youth Risk Behavior Survey 1995. Preliminary data. JAMA 1991;266:2811-12.
   Berg F. Harmful weight loss practices widespread among adolescents. HWJ/Obesity & Health 1992;6:4:69-72.
4. Youth Risk, *see 3.*
5. The Dietary Guidelines for Americans, 4th Edition, 1995. Consumer Information Center, Pueblo, CO.
   Berg F. New guidelines given for "healthy weight." Healthy Weight Journal May/Jun 1996;10:3:44, 53-54, 57.
6. JAMA 1994;272;15:11696-1202.
   Berg F. Weight loss campaign heats up. 1995;9:1:4, 11-12, 18-19.
7. Weight the Options. 1995, Natl Academy Press, Wash., DC.
   Berg F. Review: Weighing the Options. Healthy Weight Journal May/Jun 1995;9:3:57-58.
8. NIH Technology Assessment Conference: Methods for Voluntary weight loss and control. 1992.

Chapter 2
1. Newsweek. Feb 1, 1993, 64-65.
   Berg F. Gaunt idols. HWJ/Obesity & Health Mar/Apr 1993;7:2:23.
2. Fallon P, M Katzman, S Wooley, edits. Feminist perspectives on eating disorders. 1994. Guilford Press, NY.
   Health Risks of Weight Loss, 1995;89. Healthy Weight Journal, Hettinger, ND.
3. Eating Disorders 1993;1:1:52-61.
   Berg F. Television ads promote dieting. HWJ/Obesity & Health Nov/Dec 1993;7:6:106.
4. Kilbourne J. Still killing us softly: Advertising and the obsession with thinness. Fallon, *see 2.*
5. I J Eating Disorders 1992; 11:1:85-89.
   Berg F, Thin mania turns up pressure. HWJ/Obesity & Health Sep/Oct 1992;6:5:83.
   Health Risks of Weight Loss, 1995;90. Healthy Weight Journal, ND.
6. Morgan L. Why are girls obsessed with their weight? Seventeen Nov. 1989;118-119, 145, 150, 154.
7. Reported from New Scientist by Am Anorexia/Bulimia Assoc Newsletter Spring 1994;8.
   Berg F. Health Risks of Weight Loss, 1995;92. Healthy Weight Journal, ND.
8. Oswalt R, J Davis. Societal influences on a thinner body size in children. Proceedings and abstracts of the annual meeting of the Eastern Psychological Association. Philadelphia, PA. April 1990.
9. Eating Disorder Awareness Week Kit: Celebrating our natural sizes. 1996, National Eating Disorder Information Centre, Toronto.
10. Eating Disorders 1993;1:2:109-114.
    Berg F. False media messages. HWJ/Obesity & Health Jan/Feb 1994;8:1:5.
11. Nutr Forum Sep/Oct 1989, from Pediatrics 1989 83:393-397.
    Berg F. Weight Terror. HWJ/Obesity & Health Jan 1990;4:1:1.
12. Morgan L. Why are girls obsessed with their weight? Seventeen Nov. 1989;118-119, 145, 150, 154.
13. Grange D, J Tibbs, J Selibowitz. Eating attitudes, body shape, and self-disclosure in a community sample of adolescent girls and boys. Eating Dis 1995:3:3:253-264.
14. Crisp A. Anorexia nervosa in a young male. In Treating Eating Disorders, J Werne, edit. Jossey-Bass Inc, San Francisco. 1996:6.
15. Smolak L, M Levine. Toward an empirical basis for primary prevention of eating problems with elementary school children. Eat Disorders 1994;2:4:293-307.
16. Food Nutr News 1993;65:1:4.
    Berg F. Health Risks of Weight Loss, 1995;92. Healthy Weight Journal, ND.
17. Gustafson-Larson, AM, RD Terry. Weight-related behaviors and concerns of fourth-grade children. J of the Am Dietetic Assoc 1992:818-822.
18. Nichter M, S Park, M Nichter, Body image and weight concerns among African American and white adolescent females. Anthro. Dept, U of Arizona, Tucson, AZ.
    Berg F. Beauty ideas are fluid. Healthy Weight Journal Mar/Apr 1995;9:2:26.
    Health Risks of Weight Loss, 1995;123. Healthy Weight Journal, ND.
19. Young, Mary Evans. Diet Breaking: Having it all without having to diet. Hodder and Stoughton. London. 1995:5-9.
20. Rothblum E. I'll die for the revolution but don't ask me not to diet. 1994;53-76.

Fallon, *see 2.*

Berg F. Health Risks of Weight Loss, 1995; 91. Healthy Weight Journal, ND.

21. Meletiche. NAAFA News Sept/Oct 1991:5. Meletiche L. Barbie: Symbol of oppression. HWJ/Obesity & Health Sep/Oct 1993;7:5:96.

22. Smolak L, M Levine. The role of parents in the prevention of disordered eating. NEDO Newsletter 1994;17:3:1-9.

23. Levine P. President's message. Eating Disorders Awareness and Prevention Newsletter. Spring 1995:1-3.

24. Tolman D, E Debold. Conflicts of body and image, 301-317.
Fallon, *see 2.*

25. Wolf N. The beauty myth: how images of beauty are used against women, 1991. Morrow, NY.

26. Larkin J, C Rice and V Russell. Slipping through the cracks: sexual harassment, eating problems, and the problem of embodiment. Eat Disorders 1996;4:1:5-26.

27. *See 26.*

28. Levine P. The Last Word. Eat Disorders 1995;3:1:92-95.

Chapter 3

1. Niven C, D Carroll. The Health psychology of women. Harwood Academic Publ., Chur, Switzerland. 1993:115.

2. JADA 1992;92;92:7:851-53.
Berg F. Kids fear being fat early. HWJ/Obesity & Health May/June 1993;7:3:46-47.

3. Reiff D, KK Lampson Reiff, Eating Disorders: Nutrition Therapy in the Recovery Process, 1992. Aspen, Gaithersburg, MD; Personal communication with Dan Reiff, 1996.

4. Estes L, M Crago, C Shisslak. Eating disorders prevention. The Renfrew Perspective, 1996;2:1:3-5.
Fallon, *see Ch2:2.*
Berg, *see 2.*

5. Restaurants USA 1994;14:18-21.
Berg, F. Customers want bigger meals Healthy Weight Journal Mar/Apr 1995;9:2:26.

6. Taste, Health, and the Social Meal. Special issue. Journal of Gastronomy. Winter/Spring 1993.
Berg F. Review of special issue. Healthy Weight Journal May/Jun 1994;8:3:59.

7. Smolak, *see Ch2:15.*

8. Fallon, *see Ch2:2.*

9. Reiff, *see 3,* p163.

10. Nutrition News 1988;51:2:5-7.
Berg F. Weight-loss programs for children and adolescents. HWJ/Obesity & Health Oct 1989;3:10:78.

Chapter 4

1. Alexander-Mott L DB Lumsden. Understanding Eating Disorders. Taylor & Francis, Washington, DC 1994:290.

2. *See 1.*

3. *See 1.*

4. Berg F. Eating disorders — physical and mental effects. Healthy Weight Journal Mar/Apr 1995;9:2:27-30.

5. Sesan R. Feminist inpatient treatment for eating disorders. In Feminist Perspectives, p251.

6. Hoek H. The distribution of eating disorders. In Eating Disorders and Obesity, edit K Brownell and C Fairburn. Guilford Press, NY. 1995:207-211.

7. Position of the American Dietetic Association: Nutrition intervention in the treatment of anorexia nervosa, bulimia nervosa, and binge eating.

8. Wilson, GT. The controversy over dieting. Guilford Press, NY 1995:87-92.

9. Reiff, *see Ch3:3,* p312.

10. *See 9.*

11. Allis Tim, et al. Weight and See. People 1/31/94; p 50-58.

12. *See 7.*

13. Berning J, S Steen. Sports Nutr for the 90s. 1991:156-158. Aspen, Gaithesburg, MD.

14. Are (Were) You like me? The Healthy Weigh 1995;1:1:3.

15. Eating Disorder Awareness Week Kit: Celebrating our natural sizes.

16. *See Ch3:3.*

17. *See Ch3:3,* p245.

18. *See Ch3:3.*
Kaplan A, P Garfinkel. Medical issues and the eating disorders. 1993. Brunner/Mazel, NY.
Berg F. Health Risks of Weight Loss, 1995;57-58, Healthy Weight Journal, ND.
Berg F. Eating disorders affect both the mind and body. Healthy Weight Journal Mar/Apr 1995;9:2:27-30.

19. Berg F. Competitive bodybuilding. Healthy Weight Journal May/Jun 1996;10:3:47-48.

20. Wooley S. Recognition of Sexual Abuse: Progress and Backlash. Schwartz M, L Cohn, editors. Sexual abuse and eating disorders. 1996. Brunner/Mazel, New York.

21. Brewerton T. Sexual and physical assault are

risk factors for bulimia nervosa. NEDO Newsletter 1994;7:4:1-5.
22. Fallon, *see Ch2:2.*
23. Levenkron Steven, One man's experience treating a woman's disorder. Renfrew Perspective 1995;1:2:1-15.
24. *See Ch4:11,* p50-58.

Chapter 5
1. Nutrition News 1988;51:2:5-7.
    Berg F. Weight-loss programs for children and adolescents, Criteria for evaluating clinical programs. HWJ/Obesity & Health Mar 1989;3:10:78.
2. Eating and Its Disorders, edit Albert J. Stunkard and Eliot Stellar, 1984, Raven Press, NY. p 175.
3. Dietz, William, and Nevin Scrimshaw. Potential advantages and disadvantages of human obesity, from Social Aspects and Beach Publ. Luxembourg.
4. Brownell Kelly, C Fairburn. Eating Disorders and Obesity. 1995. Guilford Press, N.Y. p 417-421.
5. Stunkard A, Wadden T. Psychopathology and obesity. Human Obesity, Eds. Wurtman T, J. NY Academy of Sci 1987:57.
6. Report on Size Discrimination, NEA, 1994. For more information, contact: Mary Faber, NEA, 1201 16th St., NW, Washington, DC 20036-3290 (202-822-7700; Fax 202-822-7578.
7. Johnson C A, Self-Esteem Comes in All Sizes. 1995:8-10, Doubleday, N.Y.
8. Erdman, C K. Nothing to Lose: A Guide to Sane Living in a Larger Body. 1995. HarperCollins, N.Y.
9. Mayer K. Real Women don't Diet. 1993:115-116. Bartleby Press, Silver Spring, MD.
10. Brownell, *see 4.*
11. Hall L. Full Lives: Women who have freed themselves from food & weight obsession. 1993. Gurze Books, Carlsbad, CA.
12. Goodman C. The Invisible Woman: Confronting Weight Prejudice in America. 1995:ix-xi. Gurze Books, Carlsbad, Calif.

Chapter 6
1. Troiano R, K Flegal, et al. Overweight prevalence and trends for children and adolescents. Arch Pediatr Adolesc Med. 1995;149:1085-1091.
2. Shear C, D Freedman, et al. The Bogalusa Heart Study. Am J Public Health 1988;78:75-77.
3. Morrison J, et al. Mothers in black and white households: the NHLBI growth and health study. An J Pub Health 1994;84:1761-1767.
    Obarzanek E, G Schreiber, P Crawford, et al. Energy intake and physical activity in relation to indexes of body fat: the National Heart, Lung, and Blood Institute.
    Obarzanek E, G Schreiber, P Crawford, et al. Energy intake and physical activity in relation to indexes of body fat: the National Heart, Lung and Blood Institutes.
4. Pediatric Nutrition Surveillance System (PedNSS), Division of Nutrition, Centers for Disease Control in Atlanta.
    Berg F. High rates of childhood obesity seen in assistance programs; Overweight hits 10-year high. HWJ/Obesity & health Mar/Apr 1992;6:2:26-27, 34.
5. Berg F. Prevalences of obesity rises for minorities. HWJ? Obesity & health Jul/Aug 1993;7:4:72.
6. Fontvieille, A M and E Ravussin. Metabolic Rate and body composition Indian and Caucasian children, Critical Rev in Food Sci and Nutr 1993;33(4/5):363-368.
7. Becque MD, K Hattori, et. al. Em J Phys Anthro 71;423-249.
    Berg F. Health Risks of Obesity. 1993;4. Healthy Weight Journal, ND.
8. Bouchard C, F Johnston. Fat distribution during growth and later health outcomes. 1988. Alan Liss, NY.
    Berg F. Health Risks of Obesity 1993;43. Healthy Weight Journal, ND.
    Berg F. Ethnic differences in fat patterning. HWJ/International Obesity Newsletter Dec 1988;2:12:5.
9. Lohman T, S Gonig, et al. Concept of chemical immaturity in body composition estiamtes. Am J Hum Biol 1989;1:201-204.
10. Arch Pediatr Adolesc Med 1995;149
11. Bourch C, L Perusse, et al. Inheritance of the amount and distribution of human body fat. Int J Obesity 1988;12:205-215
    Berg F. NAASO highlights. HWJ/Obesity & Health 1992:6:1:5.
12. Mayer J. Genetic factors in human obesity. Ann NY Acad Sci 1965;131:412-421, Mayer 1965, PubEd wkshop report, p27.
13. Kumanyika S. Epidemiologic Reviews 1987;9:31-50.
    Wendorf M, I Goldfine, Diabetes 1991;40:161-165.
    Berg F. Thrifty gene may set stage for obesity in blacks, HWJ/Obesity & Health Jan/

Feb 1991:5:1:6-7.

Berg F. Former big game hunters succumb to diabetes, HWJ/Obesity & Health Nov/Dec 1991;5:6:98.

Berg F. Thrifty gene threatens the good life, Healthy Weight Journal Jul/Aug 1995;9:4:64.

14. Obarzanek, see 3.

15. Klesges Robert, J Applied Behavior Analysis, Winter 1983.

HWJ/International Obesity Newsletter Jan 1987.

16. Johnson S, L Birch. Parents' and children's adiposity and eating style. Pediatrics 1994;94:653-661.

17. J Am Diet A 1991 Sp191:9:A-81.

Berg F. Family communication. HWJ/Obesity & Health Mar/Apr 1992;6:2:24.

Berg F. Infants and young children, family tendencies hold strong influence. HWJ/Obesity & Health Dec 1989;3:12:89, 91-92, 94.

18. Mogan J, Int J Nurs Stud 1986;23:3:255-264.

19. Crawford P, L Shapiro. How obesity develops: A new look at nature and nurture. HWJ/Obesity & Health 1991;5:3:40-41.

Berg F. Fat cells: An increase in number or in size? HWJ/Obesity & health Aug 1988;2:8:1-2.

20. Filer L J. Summary of the Workshop on Child and Adolescent Obesity, University of Critical Reviews in food Science and Nutrition 1993:33:4/5:287-305.

21. See 20.

22. Giblin W P. JADA 1984;436-438.

23. Epidemiologic Reviews 1987;9:31-50.

Berg, see 13.

24. NIH Strategy Development Workshop for Public Education on Weight and Obesity, sponsored by the National Heart, Lung and Blood Institutes in 1992, p51.

25. Tufts U Diet & Nutr Ltr Jan 1993;1-2.

Berg F. Teen obesity increases heart risk. HWJ/Obesity & Health Mar/Apr 1993;7:2:31.

26. Smoak C, G Burke, et al. Relation of obesity to clustering of risk factors in children. A J of Epidemiology 1987;125:3:364-372.

Berg F. Health Risks of Obesity. 1993;24. Healthy Weight Journal, ND.

27. Mellin 1986.

Johnston 1985.

Berg F. Obesity in children and teens. HWJ/International Obesity Newsletter 1986;pilot:8:1-2

28. Frisch R, Edit. Adipose Tissue and Reproduction, 1990, Karger, Basel, Switzerland.

Berg F. High body fat brings early puberty. HWJ/Obesity & Health 1990;4:10:73-76.

Berg F. Health Risks of weight Loss. 1995:54. Healthy Weight Journal, ND.

29. Frisch, see 28.

Berg F. Health Risks of Weight Loss. 1995:51-53. Healthy Weight Journal, ND.

30. Critical Review Food Sci and Nutr 1993;93(4/5);423-430.

31. PubEd, see 24, p35.

32. Conference on the Prevention of Obesity. NIDDK, 1993:64. Abstracts:64.

33. Powers, see 24, p52.

Chapter 7

1. National Center for Health Statistics, NHANES III. Advance Data Nov 14, 12994.

Third Report on Nutrition Monitoring in US, 1995, USDA.

2. What and where our children eat: 1994 Nationwide Survey results. USDA News release, Apr 18, 1996.

3. Eaton S B, M Konner. Paleoplithic. NEJM 1985;312:5:283-289.

4. Kretchmer N, J Beard, S Carlson. The role of nutrition in the development of normal cognition. Am J Clin Nutr 1996;63:997S-1001S.

5. Levine P. Connections in primary prevention. The Renfrew Perspective Fall 1995;1:3:5-6.

6. AMA Statement, Sept 29, 1992.

7. Pollitt E. Does breakfast make a difference in school? JADA 1995;95:10:1134-1139.

8. Nicklas T. Dietary studies of children: The Bogalusa Heart Study. JADA 1995;95:1127-1133.

9. Sallis, J F. Epidemiology of physical activity and fitness in children and adolescents, Crit Rev in Food Sci and Nutr 1993;33(4/5):403-408.

10. Iverson, et al, Public Health Reports, 1985;100(2):212.

11. See 10.

12. Troiano, see Ch6:1.

13. The physically underdeveloped child, 1984: 0-438-699. USHHS, President's Council on Physical Fitness, Washington, DC.

14. Melpomene J Fall 1993;14-18, 19-26.

Berg F. Why teenage girls drop out of sports. HWJ/Obesity & Health Jan/Feb

1994;8:1:13.
15. Kratina K. Exercise dependence. 1995. Eds: K King Helm, B Klawitte. Nutrition Therapy: Advanced counseling skills. In press.
16. Berg F. Health Risks of Weight Loss. 1995;24-38. Healthy Weight Journal, ND.
17. Garner D, L Rosen. Eating disorders among athletes. J Applied Sport Sci Research 1991;5:2:100-107.
    Berg F. Health Risks of Weight Loss. 1995;55. Healthy Weight Journal, ND.
18. Wisconsin Interscholastic Athletic Association, 41 Park Ridge Drive, PO Box 267, Stevens Point, WI 54481; 715Ä344Ä8580.

Chapter 8
1. Dieting and purging behavior in black and white high school students. JADA 1992;92:3:306-312.
    Adolescents dieting. JAMA 1991;266:2811-2812.
    Berg F. Harmful weight loss practices are widespread among adolescents. HWJ/Obesity & Health Jul/Aug 1992;6:4:69-72.
2. Berg F. The weight loss industry. Regulation is needed. HWJ/Obesity & Health Jun 1990;4:6:41-46.
3. See 2.
4. JAMA 1991;266:2811-2812.
    Berg, see 1.
    JADA 1992;92:3:306-312.
5. Berg F. Health Risks of Weight Loss. 1995;50-55. Healthy Weight Journal, ND.
6. Garner, see Ch7:17.
7. Wisconsin, see Ch7:18.
8. Steen S, S McKinney. Nutrition assessment of college wrestlers. Phys Sportsmed 1986;14:100-116.
    Berg F. Weight cycling; crash dieting drops metabolism for wrestlers; Wrestling with weight. HWJ/Obesity & Health Feb 1989;3:2:1-4.
    Berg F. Health Risks of Weight Loss. 1995;52. Healthy Weight Journal, ND.
9. JAMA 191;266:2811-2812.
    JADA 1992;92:3:306-312.
    Berg, see 1.
10. Kaplan A, P Garfinkel. Medical issues and the Eating Disorders. 1993. Brunner/Mazel, New York.
11. Berg F. The case against PPA. HWJ/

Obesity & Health 1991;5:1:9-12.
12. Berg F. Weight Loss Quackery and Fads, 1995:16. Healthy Weight Journal, Hettinger, ND.
13. FDA Consumer, May 1995;3;
14. See 13.
15. Mayer, see Ch5:9, p149.
16. Hall, see Ch5:11, p96-97.
17. Rand C, A MacGregor. Adolescents having obesity surgery. Southern Med J, 1994;87:12:1208-1213.
18. Bloomers T, Exec Mgr Am Society for Bariatric Surgery, interview 1994;5.
19. Food & Nutr News Nov/Dec 1989;61:5
    Berg F. Summer weight loss camps: Not a quick fix for overweight teens. HWJ/Obesity & Health Mar 1990;4:3:29.
20. AP Feb 27, 1991.
21. JADA 1992;92:3:306-312.
    Berg, see 1.
22. Baker D and A, R Sansone. Overview of eating disorders. 1994. NEDO.
    Berg F. Health Risks of Weight Loss. 1995;40. Healthy Weight Journal, ND.
23. Mehler P, K Weiner. Frequently asked medical questions about eating disorder patients. Eating Disorders, 1994;2:1:22-30.
24. Kaplan, see Ch4:18.
25. Nutrition Labeling Watch, 1995;12.
26. Berg F. Bee pollen "cures" truckers of obesity, tumors, radiation. HWJ/Obesity & Health Mar/Apr 1991;5:2:30.
27. Rosencrans K. Diet pills suspected in deaths. Healthy Weight Journal Jul/Aug 1994;8:4:68.
28. JADA 1992;92:3:306-312.
    Berg, see Ch8:1.
29. JADA, see 28.
    Berg F. Health Risks of Weight Loss. 1995;39. Healthy Weight Journal, ND.
30. Kaplan, see Ch4:18, p101-122.
31. Clin Psych Rev 1991;11:729-780.
    Berg F. Nondiet movement gains strength. HWJ/Obesity & Health Sep/Oct 1992;6:5:85-90.
32. Satter E. How to Get Your Kid to Eat, but no too much. 1987. Bull Publ., Palo Alto, CA.
33. Smolak, see Ch2:22.
34. Reiff, see Ch3:3, p162.
35. Eating Disorder Awareness Week Kit: Celebrating our natural sizes. 1996, National Eating Disorder Information Centre, Toronto.
36. Young M Evans. Diet Breaking: Hav-

ing it all without having to diet. Hodder and Soughton, London. 1995;41-42, 56-57.

37. Obesity Research 1993;1:1:51-56.
Berg F. Linking gallstones with weight loss. HWJ/Obesity & Health May/Jun 1993;7:3:45.

38. Weighing the Options, see Ch1:7.

39. Healthy People 2000, USDHHS, PHS, Sep 1990;140.

40. NEJM 1995;333:1165-1170, 1214-1216.
Berg F. Smoking cessation impacts weight. Healthy Weight Journal Mar/Apr 1996;10:2:27-28.

41. Berg F. Smoking cessation impacts weight. HWJ 1996;10:2:27-28.

42. Healthy People 2000 1990:147.

43. Williamson D, R Anda, G Giovino, T Byers, CDC, J Madans, Kleinman. Weight gain caused by cessation of smoking. Natl Ctr for Health Statistics. 1993;324:739-745.
NEJM, see 40.
Berg F. Smokers who quit gain to average. HWJ/Obesity & Health Nov/Dec 1991;5:6:92.

Chapter 9

1. Healthy communities, healthy youth. Search Institute, 7000 S 3rd St, #210, Minneapolis, MN 55415 (1-800-888-7828, Fax 612-376-8956).

2. Berg F. Nutritionists call for new approach. HWJ/Obesity & Health May/Jun 1991;5:3:36.

3. Vitality Leader's Kit. 1994. Health Services and Promotion, Health and Welfare Canada, Ottawa.

Chapter 10

1. Healthy communities, see Ch9:1.

2. Hans, C, RD, D Nelson. A parent's guide to children's weight. 1994. N Central Regional Extension Publication 374, Iowa State Extension Service, Iowa State University of Science and Technology, Ames, Iowa 50011.

3. Fortin S, Supporting adolescents with eating problems: Suggestions for the family. National Eating Disorder Information Centre Bulletin. 1995;10:2:1-4.

4. Pediatrics 1968;41:18-29.

5. Satter E. Internal regulation and the evolution of normal growth as the basis for prevention of obesity in childhood. J Am Diet Assoc. In press.

6. Pediatrics 1994;94:654-661.

7. Crawford P, MPH RD, L Shapior, DrPH, RD. How obesity develops: a new look at nature and nurture. HWJ/Obesity & Health May/Jun 1991;5:3:40-41.

8. Satter E. The new paradigm of trust. Healthy Weight Journal Nov/Dec 1995;9:6:107-108.

9. *Ellyn Satter, MS, MSSW, RD.* How to Get Your Kid to Eat . . . But Not Too Much, *and* Child of Mine: Feeding with Love and Good Sense.

10. Johnson S, L Birch. Parents' adiposity and childrens's adiposity and eating style. Pediatrics 1994;94:653-660.

11. Ikeda J et al. Two approaches to adolescent weight reduction. J Nutr Educ 1982;14:90-92.

12. Ikeda J. Winning weight loss for teens. 1989. Bull Publishing, Palo Alto, CA.

13. 1990 Report on Television. Northbrook, IL: A.C. Nielsen Co., 1990.

14. Natl Assoc to Advance Fat Acceptance. Sacramento, CA.

15. Ikeda J, MA, RD, E Peck, DPH, RD. California takes action on children weight concerns. HWJ/Obesity & Health 1991;5:3:39.

16. Ikeda J P, MA, RD. Nutrition Education Specialist, Cooperative Extension, Dept. of Nutritional Sciences, University of California, Berkeley,. She is the author of If My Child is Too Fat, What Should I do About it?

17. J Soc Clin Psych 1985;3:425-445.

18. I J Eat Disorders 1986;5:335-346.

19. Diag/Stat Manual IIIR, Am Psychiatric Assoc 1988.

20. Bruch. Eating Disorders. Basic Books, 1973.

21. Satter E, MS, MSSW, RD. Childhood obesity demands new approaches. HWJ/Obesity & Health 1991;5:3:42-43.

22. Reprinted from HWJ/Obesity & Health 1991.

23. Johnson C. 1995. Reprinted with permission from materials compiled by Largely Positive, Inc.

24. Carol Johnson, MA. Self Esteem Comes in All Sizes. 1995.

Chapter 11

1. Allensworth D, L Kolbe. Comprehensive school health program. J School Hlth1987 57;10:409-412.
2. Wisconsin, *see Ch7:18.*
3. Project SPARK, March 1995. For more information contact: Judy Folkenberg, NIH Healthline, National Institutes of Health, Building 31, Room 2B10, Bethesda, MD 20892, 301-496-1766.
4. *See 3.*
5. *See 3,* p6-7.
6. Food & Nutrition News Mar/Apr 1995:67:2:1-4.
7. Johnston J, P Marmet, et al. Kansas LEAN: an effective coalition for nutrition education and dietary change. J Nutr Ed 1996;28:2:115-118.
8. Sallis J. Strategy Development Workshop for Public Education on Weight, NHLBI, Sept 1992.
9. Estes L, M Crago, C Shisslak. Eating Disorders Prevention. The Renfrew Perspective. 1996;2:1:3-5.
10. Piran N. On prevention and transformation. The Renfrew Perspective. 1996;2:1:8-9.

Chapter 12
1. Vitality, *see Ch9:3.*
2. Hans, *see Ch10:2.*
3. Satter, *see Ch10:9,* p69-70.
4. Olson R. Folly of restricting fat in the diet of children. Nutrition Today 1995;30:6:234-245.
5. Johnston G. New vision for exercise. HWJ/Obesity & Health Nov/Dec 1992;6:6:108.
6. Sallis J, PhD, San Diego State University, project leader, SPARK, Sports Play and Active Recreation for Kids, an ongoing research project funded by the National Institute of Health's National Heart, Lung and Blood Institute.
7. Jaffee L, P Wu. After-school activities and self-esteem in adolescent girls. Melpomene J, summer 1996;15:2:18-25; Shape Nov. 1995.
8. JADA 1995;95:1414-1417.
   Berg F. Avoid weight loss focus. Healthy Weight Journal 1996;10:4:75.
9. Melpomene J Fall 1993; 14-26.
   Berg F. Why teenage girls drop out of sports. HWJ/Obesity & Health Jan/Feb 1994;8:1:13.

10. Ryan J. The red flags of over-training. Shape Apr 1996;122-123.
11. Dwyer E, D Silbiger. The red flags of over-training. Shape Apr 1996;122.
12. Muscle & Fitness. Feb 1996:137-38, 221-2.

Chapter 13
1. Huon G. Health promotion and the prevention of dieting-induced disorders. Eat Disorders 1996;4:1:27-32.
2. NEA, *see Ch5:6.*
3. Larkin J, C Rice, V Russell. Slipping through the cracks: sexual harassment, eating problems, and the problem of embodiment. Eat Disorders 1996;4:1:5-26.
4. Pipher M. Reviving Ophelia: Saving the selves of adolescent girls. 1994. Ballantine Books, NY.

Chapter 14
1. Berg F. Health Risks of Weight Loss, 1995;122-132. Healthy Weight Journal, ND.
2. Am J Clin Nutr 1994;60:153-156.
   Berg F. Is drug abuse the next miracle cure? Healthy Weight Journal Sep/Oct 1994;8:5:84.

Chart references

Chapter 1
1. Berg F. Children in weight crisis. Healthy Weight Journal 10:5:86-87.
2. See 1.

Chapter 3
1. Garner and Garfinkel's Eating Attitudes Test, Children's version, by Maloney et. al. J Am Academy Chi Adol Psychiatry 1988;27:542-54.
   Allison D. Handbook of Assessment Methods for Eating Behaviors and Weight-Related Problems 1995;488-489. Sage Publ. Thousand Oaks, CA.

Chapter 4
1. Diagnostic criteria for eating disorders. Diagnostic and Statistical Manual, Fourth Edit. 1994. American Psychiatric Assoc., Washington, DC.
2. NEDO materials. National Eating Disorders Organization, 6655 S Yale Ave, Tulsa, OK 74136.

Chapter 6
1. Troiano R, et al. Overweight prevalence and trends for children and adolescents. Arch Pediat Adolesc Med 1995;149:1085-1091.
2. See 1.
3. See 1.
4. See 1.
5. Bouchard C, F Johnston. Fat distribution during growth and later health outcomes. 1988. Alan Liss, New York.
   Berg F. Ethnic differences in fat patterning. HWJ/Obesity & Health Dec 1988;2:12:5.
   Berg F. Health Risks of Obesity. 1995;43. Healthy Weight Journal, ND.
6. Klesges R. J Applied Behavior Analysis. Winter 1983.

Chapter 7
1. Third Report on Nutrition Monitoring in US. 1995. USDA. National Center for Health Statistics, NHANES III.
2. USHHS NHANES III. 1988-91 Advance data, NCHS, MMW, Nov 14, 1994. See 1.
3. U.S. Youth Risk Behavior Survey 1995, preliminary analysis.

Chapter 8
1. King A. A doctor's weight loss education.

HWJ/Obesity & Health guest editorial Nov/Dec 1993;7:6:104.
2. Dieting and purging behavior in black and white high school students. JADA 1992;92:3:306-312.
   Berg F. Harmful weight loss practices are widespread among adolescents. HWJ/Obesity & Health Jul/Aug 1992;6:4:69-72.

Chapter 9
1. See Ch1:1.
2. Vitality Leader's Kit. 1994. Health Services and Promotion, Health and Welfare Canada, Ottawa.

Chapter 10
1. Reprinted with permission from the National Eating Disorders Organization, from the NEDO Newsletter, Summer 1994;3.
   Smolak L, PhD, M Levine, PhD. Ten things parents can do to help prevent eating disorders in their children. Healthy Weight Journal Sep/Oct 1995;9:5:92. Linda Smolak, PhD and Michael P Levine, PhD, are eating disorder specialists at Kenyon College in Gambier, OH.
2. Levine M P, PhD. With permission from Ten things Men Can Do and Be to Help Prevent Eating Disorders. Newsletter of the National Eating Disorders Organization (NEDO), Apr/May 1994.
   Levine M P, PhD. Ten things Men Can Do and Be to Help Prevent Eating Disorders. Healthy Weight Journal Jan/Feb 1995;9:1:15.
3. National Eating Disorders Organization (NEDO), 445 E Granville Rd, Worthington, OH 43085.
4. Ikeda J. With permission from If My Child Is Too Fat, What Should I Do About It? Univ of California.
5. Satter E. With permission from Feeding with Love and Good Sense: Training Manual. 1995. Ellyn Satter Associates, 4226 Mandan Crescent, Madison, WI 53711.

Chapter 12
1. Dietary Guidelines for Americans. 1995. USDA, USDHHS.
2. Healthy People 2000. Midcourse Revisions. 1994. USDHHS, Public Health Service.

Index

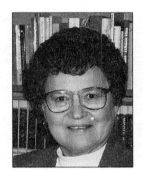 FRANCES M. BERG, M.S., LN, is the founder, publisher and editor of *Healthy Weight Journal*. A licensed nutritionist and family wellness specialist, she is the author of eight books. Berg's weekly health column, *Healthy Living,* has been published regularly in over 50 newspapers. She is Adjunct Professor at the University of North Dakota School of Medicine, Department of Community Medicine and Rural Health, Grand Forks. Her master's degree is in family social science and anthropology from the University of Minnesota.

Berg serves on the Boards of Directors of the American Diabetes Association, N.D. affiliate, and the West River Regional Medical Center. She is National Coordinator of the Task Force on Weight Loss Abuse, National Council Against Health Fraud, and a member of the Society for Nutrition Education, North American Association for the Study of Obesity, and the Society for the Study of Ingestive Behavior.

Resources for your use . . .

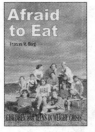

AFRAID TO EAT: Children and Teens in Weight Crisis — Today's youth are the innocent victims of society's obsession with weight — it has created a crisis of pressures to be thin, disturbed eating, stigmatization, eating disorders, and unwanted weight gain. *Afraid to Eat* brings you research, information and insight on these and other eating, weight and body image issues. Guidelines for healthful solutions for parents, teachers and health professionals; 1996, 320 pages, $21.95.

ISBN 0-918532-51-5

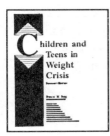

CHILDREN AND TEENS IN WEIGHT CRISIS: Summary Edition — The latest youth statistics on obesity prevalence, dieting behavior, eating disorders, fear of fat, and the stigma of overweight are at your fingertips in this new report. Guidelines call for overall child well-being, family-based programs, prevention of weight problems; 34 pages, $11.95.

ISBN 0-918532-50-7

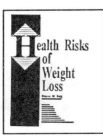

HEALTH RISKS OF WEIGHT LOSS — Winner of Outstanding Academic Book of the Year selection. A MUST-READ report for educators, health professionals, athletic trainers and the dieting public. This book documents the risks of dieting, semi-starvation, weight cycling, purging, disturbed eating, diet pills; 168 pages, $21.95.

ISBN 0-918532-44-2

"Highly recommended!" - Journal of Nutrition Education

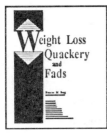

WEIGHT LOSS QUACKERY AND FADS — Quackery in diet products is at an all time high. You need to know what misinformation the public is buying. Here are the latest facts on "fat burning" pills, herbal teas, chromium picolinate, body wraps, thigh cream, and many more. How to identify and report fraud; 31 pages, $11.95.

ISBN 0-918532-60-4

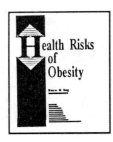
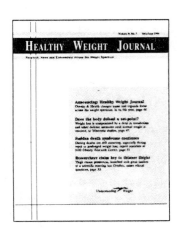

ORDER NOW
to get the facts you need!

YES! I want to receive the top resources in the field of healthy weight management. Please send me immediately the publications checked below:

☐ **Afraid to Eat: Children and Teens in Weight Crisis** — **$21.95**

☐ **Children and Teens in Weight Crisis: Summary Edition** — **$11.95**

☐ **Health Risks of Obesity** — **$29.95**

☐ **Health Risks of Weight Loss** — **$21.95**

☐ **Weight Loss Quackery and Fads** — **$11.95**

☐ **Healthy Weight Journal** — **$59.00/year** (bimonthly)

NAME --

ADDRESS ---

TELEPHONE ---

Total $_____

Method of payment US funds only :
☐ Enclosed
☐ Bill me Institutions only PO#_____
☐ Visa
☐ MasterCard

Card # _ _ _ _ _ _ _ _ _ _ _ _ _ _ _ _

Exp. date_____

Signature_____

POSTAGE
BOOKS: U.S.–$3.00 1st book, $1 each additional; Foreign–$3.00 surface each; $9.00 airmail. SUBSCRIPTIONS: Foreign – add $5.00/year.

Guarantee: Your satisfaction 100% guaranteed or receive a full refund, no questions asked.

FAX TO **701-567-2602** OR CALL **701-567-2646**

HEALTHY WEIGHT JOURNAL, 402 SOUTH 14TH STREET, HETTINGER, ND 58639